EMOTIONAL
BALANCE

EMOTIONAL BALANCE

The Path to Inner Peace and Healing

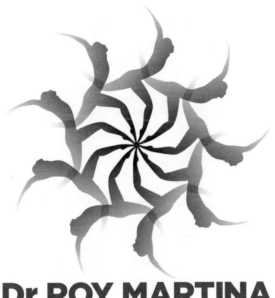

Dr ROY MARTINA

HAY HOUSE

Australia • Canada • Hong Kong • India
South Africa • United Kingdom • United States

First published and distributed in the United Kingdom by:

Hay House UK Ltd, 292B Kensal Rd, London W10 5BE. Tel.: (44) 20 8962 1230; Fax: (44) 20 8962 1239. www.hayhouse.co.uk

Published and distributed in the United States of America by:

Hay House, Inc., PO Box 5100, Carlsbad, CA 92018-5100. Tel.: (1) 760 431 7695 or (800) 654 5126; Fax: (1) 760 431 6948 or (800) 650 5115. www.hayhouse.com

Published and distributed in Australia by:

Hay House Australia Ltd, 18/36 Ralph St, Alexandria NSW 2015. Tel.: (61) 2 9669 4299; Fax: (61) 2 9669 4144. www.hayhouse.com.au

Published and distributed in the Republic of South Africa by:

Hay House SA (Pty), Ltd, PO Box 990, Witkoppen 2068. Tel./Fax: (27) 11 467 8904. www.hayhouse.co.za

Published and distributed in India by:

Hay House Publishers India, Muskaan Complex, Plot No.3, B-2, Vasant Kunj, New Delhi – 110 070. Tel.: (91) 11 4176 1620; Fax: (91) 11 4176 1630. www.hayhouse.co.in

Distributed in Canada by:

Raincoast, 9050 Shaughnessy St, Vancouver, BC V6P 6E5. Tel.: (1) 604 323 7100; Fax: (1) 604 323 2600

A catalogue record for this book is available from the British Library.

ISBN 978-1-84850-227-7

Printed in the UK by CPI William Clowes Ltd, Beccles, NR34 7TL

This paper is manufactured from material sourced from forests certified according to strict environmental, social and economical standards.

CONTENTS

ACKNOWLEDGEMENTS

I am grateful to be alive and to get the chance to learn and grow, so whoever is responsible for this, thank you, thank you, thank you.

I would like to thank all the women who have helped me grow and learn what unconditional love is. I apologize for being a slow student and still not getting it completely. Especially, I want to thank my grandmother, my mother, Erica, Marli, Patricia, Maryann, Annelot, Mayana and my three sisters: Patricia, Maritza and Annelies.

I am very grateful to have two incredibly talented sons who have incarnated to help me to the next level of evolution. Joey and Sunray, I love you more than myself.

To my dad Patricio: for sticking to the script we agreed upon before coming to Earth.

To my mother Estanita: for loving me even when I was at my worst.

For Kate: for your friendship through lifetimes.

For Marnie: my friend in good times and bad times.

For Robbie Kaman, Rick Steward, Roberto Re, Massimo Romani and Bertie Zwaans.

For Anastasia: soulmates in heaven and on Earth.

For Veronica: for your help and friendship.

For the thousands of souls who come to my workshops and read my books or have been my patients at some point in time.

I want to thank you, my reader, for picking up this book and taking the time to read my thoughts. I wish you a happy experience and may your life be blessed with health and happiness and be full of joy, grace and ease.

For my team at Roy Martina Experience, including Joop, Jose, Joke, Agnes and all those working hard to support me in bringing my concepts to the world.

Last but not least, to two special people without whose help my life would be much more complicated: Yvonne Lucardie and Fons Claessens.

PREFACE

Dear reader, this book is based on my 50-plus years of research into balancing my life, finding inner peace and being happy with myself. As you will find out, it has been a long, winding road, but eventually I have succeeded. Helping myself has also enabled me to help tens of thousands of my patients, and later on hundreds of thousands of people through this book and my workshops. This book has already been published in Dutch and was a bestseller. This improved and updated English edition contains my latest ideas, discoveries and techniques. I have discovered new ways to help heal our immortal souls, so you are in for a great journey. I have made it really easy for you and it does not require a big investment of your time, but will give you a big return in quality of life. This book offers many tools to enrich your life and heal the past. It can guide you on your path to inner peace. Read it more than once; it gives you back more each time you read it. Then start using the special Emotional Healing Formula and other Emotional Balancing exercises.

Share this knowledge with others and help each other; in the beginning and end we are all One.

Live each day as if it were your last, but with no regrets.

Do it your way, because that is the only way!

I hope we will meet somewhere in this space-time event to share our many healing stories and learn more from each other.

Wishing you a great journey, which in fact is no journey.

25 June 2010
Jupiter, Florida

INTRODUCTION

THE THREE LEVELS OF CONSCIOUSNESS

With all the doom and gloom around due to the economic crisis, at one of my recent workshops on the Law of Attraction, one participant piped up, 'It's easy for you to say that we attract what we need; you are successful and you have enough money, but that's not the case for all of us!'

I smiled and replied, 'You are absolutely right, it *is* easy for me to say, but not for the reasons you mention. Success is not what you think it is. The fact that I have 300 people in the room and you believe I make more money than you is not a measure of my success. The fact is that I attracted this group here, yes, but the question is: was it the result of luck, smart marketing or science? What I want you to believe is that a science is behind it. This science is made up of two parts: Inner and Outer. The Inner part is how I feel about myself. Do I consider myself worthy enough? Do I feel happy about what I am doing? Do I feel that by doing what I am doing I am giving something of value to the participants? The Outer is the marketing, the brochures and the website. I might be able to fool a lot of people with just the Outer part, but they would never come back and would leave dissatisfied with the workshop, if my Inner work did not match their expectations. When my Inner matches my Outer and both are aligned in positive energy, my success will increase and be consistent. Word of mouth is the best marketing that exists.

In the end it is not about money, it is about being happy being you. Do you accept where you are right now? Have you decided to take more control of your future, or are you just going to wait and see if your luck changes? If what you have is not what you want, then you have to do everything you can to change so you will attract more of what you want. And then you keep doing that, changing your strategies until you have manifested what you want. I am willing to do what is necessary. Are you? If the answer is yes,

I can teach you how. The end result is always the ultimate success: being happy with who you are, where you are and what you have, and who you share it with.'

The workshop participant looked at me and said simply, 'Thank you!'

We all have one thing in common: we want to be happy. Happiness can mean a roof over your head, enough to eat, healthy children or a happy relationship. Some people seek a higher form of happiness, sometimes known as 'bliss'. Bliss is what I refer to as the highest expression of happiness.

In order to reach a state of bliss and maintain this, we need to distinguish between three levels of happiness.

Level 1: Competitive Happiness

This we see in sport, business, war, games, gambling, school, etc. *We feel happy when we win and are ahead of others.* This form of happiness is always transient, however, and may sooner or later turn against us. Some people get stuck at this level and can become very unhappy and destructive when they lose.

Level 2: Conditional Happiness

This kind of happiness can be seen when we are very happy when we are young, strong, good-looking and full of energy, and become depressed when the symptoms of old age set in. We are happy when a child is born and become unhappy when that child turns into a hyperactive, uncontrollable brat or gets to puberty and rebels against us. We are happy with our friends as long as they are nice to us but not when they tell us something we don't want to hear. When we fall in love everything is fantastic, until a few years later when we are more critical. Conditional happiness never lasts and sooner or later we discover that things were not as we thought they were and we become unhappy with what we have.

Level 3: Unconditional Happiness

With this level of happiness, we need no outside stimulus to feel happy or at peace.

We have accepted the fact that we are fallible mortal human beings, we accept and welcome change, death and suffering. We are comfortable with both discomfort and pleasure, and are not attached to outcomes, but enjoy the process of experiencing life to its fullest. We are grateful for all the blessings and experiences that we have along the way and we are at peace with ourselves and others. We let go of the need to judge or be right, and we forgive easily. We also understand that we are one with the universe. We are, most of the time, in the turbulence-free zone that I call the still-point.

Still-point: the Place to Be

Bliss is the silence of perfection, which is the spectrum of all there is, like sunlight containing all colours. When we are in still-point we feel inner peace, harmony and love, and we know that all is good as it is, even if it is not what we want. When we are not connected to our natural state of being in harmony with ourselves and our surroundings, we feel alone, abandoned, unloved, rejected and powerless.

This book is about finding your still-point, which is about connecting to the Divine Essence in you and around you. My definition of God is bound to be limited, so in order to make this as boundless and unlimited as possible, God must be 'all': all there is, all there ever was and all that will ever be. This is what we constantly forget and neglect by disengaging from our Divine Essence. When we isolate ourselves energetically we feel small and alone. Isolation is always a self-inflicted event: we do it to ourselves and we become so good at it that we believe it has been forced upon us by others, circumstances, nature or an act of God. The main reason we forget who we really are is that we focus on our five senses, which are very limited. Our reality is a projection created by our limited senses. Because we grow up in a world where people are not aware of who they really are, we also start to believe that limitations, pain, disease and suffering are normal. Most people are unaware of their potential and keep creating patterns in their lives that indicate that they are disconnected from their inner source of power. Knowledge is passed on from generation to generation – and this becomes the greatest limitation of all. To achieve the wisdom needed to find unconditional happiness, we need to liberate ourselves from the many limiting beliefs we have grown up with. Only then can we circumvent our projected reality and get a sense of all there is.

Swarupa: Our Potential

There is a beautiful tale in Vedic literature that illustrates who we really are.

In a forest in India, a lioness gave birth to a little lion cub. The mother unfortunately died soon after, when the cub was just a few weeks old. The cub wandered off after trying to wake up his mother and got lost in the woods looking for food. By a stroke of luck he found a ewe feeding her young. He was accepted among the sheep and grew up in their company. Naturally he did not know that he was a lion. He felt weird at times because he had trouble learning to bleat and because the grass was hard for him to digest, but he did not know any better. One day, while the sheep were doing their normal grazing, a big lion came roaring and running after them. The sheep were terrified and ran away bleating – and so did the lion cub. The big lion stopped in surprise at seeing a lion cub being afraid of him and bleating like a sheep. He grabbed the lion cub in his mouth and carried it away in the jungle. The lion explained to the frightened cub that he was not going to eat him, because the cub was the son of a lion, but that it was not acceptable for lions to be in the company of sheep. The cub could not grasp what the lion was telling him and kept saying, 'Don't eat me, please!' The lion knew then that the cub was not aware of who he really was. He took him to a nearby river and made him look at his image in the reflecting water. The cub at last accepted that the lion was right. Instantly he began walking like a lion. He stopped bleating and started to roar like his fellow lions.

Most of us are exactly like this lion cub: we have forgotten our true nature. We are surrounded by others who are like sheep, and we go through life with our heads down, frightened and unable to recognize the strong and noble creature within. This tale speaks to the divine spark we all carry within us, also known as the Higher Self.

We Are Divine Beings

Once we accept and act upon our divinity with single-minded certainty, we will become masters of our destiny and live with self-respect, facing the challenges of our path boldly. We will treat everyone as equally divine even when they are not aware of it. Only then will it become effortless for us to overcome anger, hatred, jealousy and greed, and to feel instead the exuberance of love and empathy.

That's where we are going in this book: we are training and disciplining our minds gracefully and skilfully, step by step.

Free Yourself from Slavery

The question most people ask me is: 'Why do we become slaves of our own minds?' The answer will be very clear once you have read this book, but for now I would like to give you some basic principles.

In order to survive we are born with certain basic survival programs. As babies, our lives are simple: eat, sleep, excrete and grow. In order to achieve our goals we have to be loveable; for this reason babies are built to be cute and huggable. Even the sounds we make are programmed to attract attention and instil panic when needed. You cannot say this all happens consciously; it's all part of an unconscious program that each of us needs in order to make it through early life. As we grow older, we learn through appropriate training how to overcome and override this basic survival program. Parents show us affection and love even when we are not hungry and fulfil our basic needs through quality time, respect, admiration, trust, acknowledgment, understanding, acceptance, comfort, encouragement, care, approval, etc., without us having to give up anything, just for who we are. If that does not happen, however, we crave and seek to fulfil those needs.

The biggest problem is that we are programmed to find people who in general will *not* give us what we want and need.

As a consequence we get more and more desperate and become either more depressed and clingy or the opposite: bitter, aggressive, negative. We tend to blame either ourselves or the world for not getting our needs met. *The only control that works is letting go of control!*

The goal of this book is to make you aware of how this works so you can overcome this unconscious programming.

To get back to the three basic levels of consciousness, these can be classified as:

Level 1: Matter
Level 2: Energy
Level 3: Anti-matter

For anything to be formed in matter there must first be a conceptual blueprint in anti-matter, which needs to be energized and then materializes in shape and form. Let's take this concept further and look at how we create our goals, desires, dreams and wishes in our lives.

Level 1: Working Hard

Hard work uses up a great deal of energy; we often find resistance and are limited by the amount of hours in a day. At this level we find most of the motivational gurus: Anthony Robbins, Les Brown, Zig Ziglar and others.

Keyword: intensity. If you are at this level and you want to be successful, it means you are working hard and very intensely. You may be very successful, but often this success comes at a steep price. At this level, *material manifestation is the paramount goal.*

Level 2: Working Smart

Many of us arrive here after having worked hard for a long period of time, when the realization hits how futile that approach is or that it comes at too high a price. We come to the realization that if we work smarter, we can do less. We start listening to our feelings and following our intuition. *If we make choices from our gut level (intuition), we become successful in creating a harmonious life.* At this level we are more inclined to follow leaders such as Stephen Covey, Dennis Waitley and Joan Borysenko.

Keyword: intuition. If you are at this level and you want to be successful, it will mean you will be guided by your core values. Family and happiness are more important than career. The tendency here is often to settle for less than is necessary, and often there is confusion about wealth and success. If intuition and feelings are suppressed, there can be a tendency toward immune dysfunction, cancer and chronic fatigue syndrome. *Balance and harmony are essential at this level.*

Level 3: Not Working at All

'Not working' is a deceptive term; it is better to use the word 'effortlessness'. This is the path of least resistance. Work does not cost us energy but gives us a boost and energizes us. At this level we have become synchronized with the universe. We attract the right people at the right time in our lives and we create instantly. Others consider this coincidence or luck. We don't waste energy. We are completely tuned in to our higher consciousness and feel guided. We know that we are responsible for all the events in our lives. At this level we find leaders and teachers such as Deepak Chopra, Neale D. Walsh, Wayne Dyer and others. Being at this level we realize that we are all unlimited beings and that the universe is here to support us. This is the level of maximal synchronicity, the level of surrender and allowing our intentions to be manifested by the universe.

Keyword: intention. *Being of service is what it's all about at this level.* If you are at this level, success comes without strenuous efforts and you are aware of all the signals that the universe sends to you. You are in communication with your guides. Spiritual growth is your priority and you let go of all that distracts you from it. Relationships are based on spiritual values and not conditional love. You totally trust the connection with the universe. This is the level of true healing. Most of us do not succeed at keeping ourselves at this level. Also you need to realize that there are various sub-levels.

Most people are dominant in one of these levels. This does not mean that the other levels are not present. This is not about judging the work of any of the writers and thinkers mentioned; they do important work and for our evolution it is natural to start at Level 1 and move up. Nor do I say that I am at Level 3 all the time, although I certainly wish I were.

Mastery

There are many ways to look at this concept, and in the course of this book we will deal with many of them. To become skilful at anything we need to go through these three levels: first, hard work to build up a winning habit in our neurological system. In this way we go from 'unconscious incompetent' to 'conscious competent'.

Secondly, we start to work smarter; we listen to our natural rhythms and our bodies. We now start becoming what we want. We don't have to think about it anymore: we are 'unconscious competent'.

Thirdly, we have done a thing so many times that we can do it effortlessly; we are now 'unconscious excellent'. This is the level of mastery.

In order to master anything we need one ingredient: self-discipline. It is most powerful when it comes from the heart and not from the mind. Children learn to walk and, later, run because they want it badly and nothing can stop them. Some people achieve excellence at what they do because they love it; self-discipline from the heart is effortless. That's where I want to coach you, to use your emotions to develop yourself to a point of effortlessness.

Where Are You Right Now?

Before we continue, let's evaluate where you are right now. This will give us an overview of what areas to focus on.

First, I would like to recommend and encourage you to buy a journal, preferably with a hardback cover. This journal will become a guide for your journey. You can keep track of your progress. Take a few minutes every day to record what's happening. Later on we will define what your turbulence is and how you can learn to stop losing energy.

Once you have your journal, jot down your answers:

- What makes you stressed?
- What are you working hard to achieve?
- Which people annoy you the most? How do you deal with them?
- What are you most intense about?
- What costs you least effort?
- In which areas of your life do you feel you are using your intuition?
- In which areas do you not?
- What proceeds effortlessly and gives you joy?
- What are you most passionate about?
- Do you often feel connected to the universe?
- Do you like being of service to others? How do you do that, and how do you contribute to making this planet a better place?
- What are you doing to become more loving and more compassionate?
- What conclusions can you reach?

Yin Needs Yang as Yang Needs Yin

In Traditional Chinese Medicine, the two opposite (and complementary) polarities of nature are referred to as *yin* and *yang*. Yang is expansive, aggressive, male-like and externally focused energy. Yin is inward focused, softer, female-like energy. The whole yin/yang philosophy is about two opposing forces that modify the polarity of energy, also called *Chi*. When the two are balanced, a peaceful, harmonious state called Tao is created.

This has been backed up by what we now know of quantum physics. The laws of energy govern our lives and by understanding them and working with them, we create harmony and longevity.

Let's look at the three levels again:

LEVEL 1	LEVEL 2	LEVEL 3
yang	yin	Tao
conscious	subconscious	higher conscious
reason	feeling	knowing
intellect	intuition	insight
hard	smart	effortless
matter	energy	blueprint (anti-matter)
intensity	intuition	intention
brain (mind)	heart	spirit
knowledge	belief system	wisdom
competitive happiness	conditional happiness	unconditional happiness
routine	feeling state	flow state
future focus	past focus	now focus
curing	healing	loving/being
scientific	natural	magical (spontaneous)
coincidence	synchronicity	instant creation
logic-rational	intuitive	miraculous

From the Illusion of Control to the Reality of Being Guided

Here is an overview of the characteristics of the three different states. When we are at Level 1, things happen to us, we have bad luck or good luck, coincidences happen that influence our lives. At Level 2, we start seeing the connections between different events. But still we are not in control; we accept and follow the guidance we get. At Level 3, we consciously create our own reality; we are mastering the cosmic game and we are in synchronicity with the cosmic intentions. We let go of ego and surrender to the all-binding universal force.

At Level 1, we find our own way without the map of our spirit. At Level 2, we have a mobile phone and we ask for directions. At Level 3, we have a GPS that guides us effortlessly to the best and most efficient way forward.

Who Is the Creator of My Reality?

One of the questions asked most frequently on my seminars is: 'How do I get from Level 1 to Level 3?' The fastest way to get to Level 3 is via Level 2. That's the shortcut. You get to Level 2 by learning to feel and hear your inner guidance, and trusting it. There will be many roadblocks and detours on your way. Who creates them? You do! In order to grow spiritually, we need to accept a basic principle: *we create our own reality.*

In other words: nothing happens *to* you; there are no coincidences in life, there is no punishment, there is only cause and effect. This is also referred to as *karma*. We will discuss this intensively in the next section.

The moment we accept our role as creators of our own destiny, we also realize that we can create what we really want. This leads us to the next question.

What Do You Really Want?

If you are at Level 1, what you really want is *matter*. You subconsciously seek security! You want to create more matter than you could possibly need.

If you are at Level 2, what you really want is to feel good all the time, you want to be loved, get attention, get respect, get trust, get admiration, be cared for. You are nice to others because that will give you more of what you want.

If you are at Level 3, what you really want is to become one with the universe. You become of service and surrender to the highest source. You derive joy from being you, letting go of fears and making choices based on what's best for your spiritual growth. You seek conscious communion.

In this book we will constantly come back to the concept of these three levels. In all aspects of life you will find these three at work. If you want to maximize the effort you make in order to create happiness in our lives, you have to make happiness an effortless state of being. We can be sad and still be in 'bliss' when we realize that the sadness is nothing but a focal point of our awareness, and that as soon as we refocus on our being we are back in harmony and still-point.

KARMA CONSCIOUSNESS

To develop inner peace, you need to understand what upsets your spirit. So here are some points to ponder and read (and re-read) until they are 100 per cent part of your consciousness. They are your basic guidance on the path to inner peace. Karma is like yin and yang; it is either love-connected (also known as positive karma) or it is linked to ego (fear-based).

Time to Journal

Write down what resonates most with you; these are the areas that you need to work on:

- To reach inner peace, you have to get rid of your fear-based emotions and interact with your Divine Self directly.
- Karma is produced by what you think or say, and also your judgements, your motives and intent. So if you judge a person and yet say something opposite to what you are thinking, you are still creating karma. In this case your judgement is coming from your suppressed emotions and unresolved conflicts.
- Karma also means that you have attracted, manifested and so you are responsible for everything that shows up in your life. When you transcend the challenges on your path, to paraphrase Nietzsche: 'What does not kill you makes you more loving and wise!' Then you are evolving and becoming closer to your Inner Divine Power.
- Buddhism states that the cause of suffering comes from attachment and resistance. What you resist, persists and,

by giving more energy to it, it gets bigger and depletes your life-force more and more. Resistance makes us lose lots of life-force and causes disease and suffering. Unresolved conflicts create a permanent source of resistance. Doing what you resist eats up your energy. What you resist you draw to you.

- The best and fastest path to inner peace is guided meditation. With the right meditation, from day one you can go deep into a trance like someone who has been practising for 10 years or more. The goal of meditation is to be able to focus your mind on where you want it to be. In Buddhism it is said that the mind is like a hyperactive chattering monkey. Learning to calm it down will change your life.

- Avoid people who tell you that they know what is best for you. You have to find your own path. Find techniques that will bring you closer to your power.

- Assumptions and expectations are the two illusions from which you have to detach yourself. Be aware of your assumptions and expectations and know immediately that you are projecting yourself on the situation or person. You expect people to be like you or like others, and for that reason you do not see them as they really are. Don't treat people like you want to be treated; treat them the way *they* want to be treated. Practise unconditional acceptance. Every time you get upset with someone else, it is because you have expectations that are in conflict with what is.

- Guilt and blame are forms of self-pity. You need to let go of them. We are here to learn from our past but not to suffer because of it.

- Your truth is what you find inside and can change over time as you evolve and understand your immortality better. There are no rigid rules in truth; it is based on your beliefs, your power to observe, your education and how far you are to transcend those.

- When you suppress your emotions, you are blocking the flow of life itself and you will have to re-balance that karmic event sooner or later. Loving and accepting yourself even when you are vulnerable or feel weak is the first step to healing.

- Beliefs create your reality but are not *in* reality. They limit your perception and influence how you filter information. If you want to change your reality, you'd best change your beliefs.

- The best place to be at any moment is where you are in that moment. Practise being in the moment, observing and becoming a witness of life itself. Like John Lennon said, life is what happens to you while you're busy making other plans. In the now you have the most power.

- Nothing that is done or said to you is personal. The other person is projecting his or her own unresolved issues onto you. It has nothing to do with you, and would have happened to anyone else in that place at that time. What other people do does not affect you. What you *think* about what they do, however, does directly affect you.

- Your subconscious mind is the part of you driving your intentions and controlling your life. It contains a self-image that is a prison for you to live in. To break free you have to change who you believe you are and transcend your own limiting view of yourself.

- What you give you shall receive, so show mercy, grace and love; you will receive the same in return. If you want respect, become good at showing respect. If you want appreciation, become a master of appreciating others.

- The best control over any situation is to give up control and believe in yourself. You always have the free will to choose how you will respond in any situation.

- Unresolved issues become your shadow; all that you do not deal with and do not or cannot heal will pursue you relentlessly. What you leave incomplete or unresolved, you'll be doomed to repeat.

- Be patient with yourself and others. Be compassionate and generous. Accept your kindness as self-serving, and express it anyway. Engage in acts of random kindness. You will be rewarded exponentially even when you do so because you know you will be rewarded.

- Love yourself and accept your imperfections as a challenge to direct you to finding your perfection inside. Everything you require to make your life happy and fulfilling is within you.

- Forgiveness is self-liberation from past traumas and hurt. Everything you refuse to forgive in yourself and others remains with you. Karma is the law of infinite patience, as you will be given chance after chance to practise forgiveness.

- Where your attention goes, your energy flows. Attention creates your emotional reality. So if you focus on what is not good in your life, you will attract more of that. The goal is to keep your attention on what you really want and to be grateful for all that is good in your life. Count your blessings every day. The more you do that, the more you will have to be grateful for.

THE POWER OF INTENT

Intention is the starting point of everything we desire or create. Not all our intentions are conscious.

There are four levels of intention:

1. **Conscious intention: the things we desire and dream of at a conscious level.**
2. **Subconscious intention: what our subconscious mind desires and fears.**
3. **Soul's intention: to heal and balance unresolved issues, conflicts and hurts.**
4. **Spirit's intention: to evolve and get closer to ourselves so we will keep growing and getting more and more detached from the illusion of reality, and closer to our ability to love unconditionally.**

We control only at the conscious level; the goal of this book is to free yourself from any outcome and at all times connect to that space in yourself where there is no conflict but only inner peace.

It is the creative power that fulfils all of our needs, desires and dreams, whether for money, career, healing, relationships, spiritual awakening or love. Everything that happens in the universe begins with intention.

Time to Journal

As you begin this new journey, you become more aware of a path filled with unlimited possibility. Take some time to consider your intentions, your desires and where you want to focus your attention in the months ahead. The classic Vedic text the Upanishads declares, 'You are what your deepest desire is. As your desire is, so is your intention. As your intention is, so is your will. As your will is, so is your deed. As your deed is, so is your destiny.'

OUR DUALISTIC MIND

As you know, we live in a dualistic world. We have a right and left brain: the left brain is the computer that analyzes and is rational. The right brain is connected to our deeper and hidden levels. Together they create two realities: the conscious mind and the unconscious mind.

Human consciousness can be compared to an iceberg, of which the largest part (our subconscious mind) lies under the surface of the water.

Incongruence Is Duality at Work

This duality of consciousness can create congruence or incongruence. When the two parts of the mind are aligned, we are on a path of effortlessness and flow. When there is conflict we will sabotage ourselves. A good example is weight loss: no one gets excited about starting another diet. Dieting is associated with suffering and deprivation. When the conscious mind associates more pain with being overweight than with dieting, we can start a diet. This will be successful as long as one has the willpower and endurance to give up many treats. When the subconscious mind moves in to sabotage our willpower, it will succeed. This is why fewer than 6 per cent of those who diet will manage to keep the weight off permanently.

In short, change requires the unrestricted compliance and cooperation of the subconscious. In the subconscious we have our self-image and our history, including all our unresolved issues and suppressed emotions. The subconscious mind prefers the status quo or the comfort zone, even when this is not perfect.

Communicating with the Subconscious

Over the years and with the aid of a technique called kinesiology, I've found a way to communicate with the subconscious mind. Kinesiology is a system where you test a person's muscle strength while asking him or her questions. When someone is not congruent with a statement or question, the body will react with stress and muscle power will diminish for a few seconds.

As you work with the techniques in this book, you will begin to overcome many of your unconscious self-sabotaging mechanisms. I wish you a successful journey to the deeper parts of yourself, where you are already at peace and in harmony.

PART I

Emotions Are
Energy in Motion

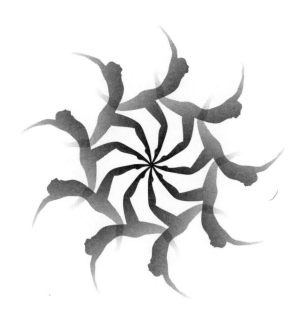

CHAPTER 1

UNRESOLVED EMOTIONS: OUR SHADOW WORLD

FREE CHOICE

In order to grasp the concept of emotional balance, we must first understand what emotions really are. The emotions we experience are based on conditioning and unconscious patterns from our past; most of the time they are not based on free choice. Free choice is a conscious decision.

We can divide our sensations into two categories: pleasant and unpleasant. We make distinctions between the kind of pleasant or unpleasant feelings we have. This normally enables us to know what to do to change the feeling. Some people focus only on feeling bad. The glass is almost always half-empty when it could also be seen as half-full.

FIRST STEP IN AWARENESS

So what are these emotions and how do they become so powerful that they can control us instead of us being in charge? How do we get to emotional balance?

Emotional intelligence is the ability to recognize, acknowledge, accept and work with your emotions in a way that does not suppress them. Emotions thus become a guiding force for survival and success. Our emotional state determines our behaviour.

Think about how you would react if you were in a traffic jam and you'd just won a considerable sum of money on the lottery. Now imagine that traffic jam after an awful night quarrelling with your partner. Would you react differently? Most of us would. Emotions are the basis of our actions.

WHAT'S KARMA GOT TO DO WITH IT?

When we talk about negative karma we should realize that most of our negative emotional reactions spring from unresolved issues from the past. By not making conscious choices based on being aligned with our highest values, we stay in a negative vicious circle. The emotions can also point us in the right direction and help us make more appropriate choices that will create positive karma. Example: a stranger (let's say someone ahead of us in the queue at the supermarket) yells at you for no reason whatsoever. How would you react? Some people might be aggressive. Others would never go to that supermarket ever again. Some people would file a complaint, others would feel bad for a long time to come. It all depends on the emotional state of mind they were in at the time. More evolved people will immediately understand that the person has issues that are not yet resolved and that it has nothing to do with them personally and will feel compassion and love for this person and may even offer their help if that is a possibility.

WHAT ARE EMOTIONS?

Emotions belong to our *heartware*, while reason belongs to our *hardware* (neurological wiring). When there is no balance between the two, there will be stress.

Emotions are almost impossible to define correctly. Emotions are often described as feelings. But is an emotion really just a feeling? According to my findings, an emotion is an *association* we have with a certain sensation. The sensation itself is often predominantly energetic in nature, coupled with electro-chemical reactions in the central nervous system. The electro-chemical reactions are secondary to the energetic reactions. Every time we experience an emotion there is a quantum of energetic build-up that needs to be released. In other words: emotion stands for energy that needs direction, irrespective of the cause. The cause or stimulus is not important at all, and can be important or irrelevant; it is what we *do* with this energy that makes all the difference.

Experiencing emotions is one side of the coin; expressing them is the other.

The problem is that it's not always practical to express our emotions.

SUPPRESSION: THE BEGINNING OF THE KARMIC CYCLE

We learn to suppress emotions early in life in order to fit the mould our parents want for us. There are different ways to suppress our emotions:

- denial (not acknowledging the feeling)
- reasoning (dissociating)
- trivializing (minimizing)
- positive thinking (can be a form of all the above)
- resistance (not accepting)
- guilt (blaming ourselves)
- overruling (replacing with other feelings).

In order to understand what happens when we suppress our emotions, we need to understand more about energy circulation. In the 5,000-year-old Chinese medical art of acupuncture, the theory is that every organ produces a specific type of energy, referred to as *Chi*. This Chi is transported to the 100 trillion-plus cells and tissues all over the body. This is done through an elaborate system known as the *meridians*. The essence of the energy is different depending on which organ produces it. Liver-energy, for example, has a distinct rate of vibration to kidney-energy.

Traditional Chinese Medicine identifies five basic elements: Fire, Earth, Metal, Water and Wood. The most interesting concept we can learn from TCM is how the emotions and organs are linked. Unresolved emotions will affect the corresponding and related organs and tissues. To translate this from acupuncture to more practical terms, let's look at some examples: prolonged and inappropriately handled frustration may lead to gallstones or gallbladder disease. There is a much higher occurrence of gallstones in obese women who have tried many diets than in obese women who have not gone on the dieting-route or other control groups.

My belief is that there may be a link to frustration. Chronic anxiety and worries will affect the stomach meridian and can lead to gastritis. According to the latest research, worries affect the immune system and thereby make us more prone to infections. Stomach ulcers are linked with a bacteria called *Helicobacter pylori* and are treated 'successfully' with antibiotics. The real cause is almost never addressed in traditional Western medicine: why are we vulnerable to *H. pylori* in the first place?

SCIENCE VERSUS EXPERIENCE

Let's assume the Eastern scientists have observed correctly the connections between emotions and energy – is there any proof to be found in Western medicine? Dr Deepak Chopra, one of the pioneers in bringing to the fore valuable ancient knowledge supported by the latest research, speaks about *the quantum mechanical body*. As discussed in his book *Perfect Health*, this is a network that responds immediately to our slightest thoughts and emotions. It is not localized in space-time but is far more general, extending in all directions like a field. You cannot see your own quantum body, but you can become aware of it. Energy follows some simple laws; one of those laws is that energy does not disappear – it changes form. It can become matter, but it cannot disappear; there will remain a memory or energy field.

Another pioneer of our times is Professor William Tiller, PhD. In his book *Science and Human Transformation*, he delves into subtle energies and consciousness. He is one of the world's leading scientists on the structure of matter and has researched homeopathy, yoga, Qigong, meditation, lasers and more. He has created a new model that takes science to a completely new level. In a later chapter we will continue with the ramifications of his work when we look at the meridians and chakras. Suffice to say that information (emotions are a form of information) will affect matter and that meridians do exist and do transport energy through our bodies. Anyone denying this is not really open to scientific advancements, but is locked up in his or her own prejudices.

KILLERS OF MEN

Let's take a look at the leading killers in Western society. Heart disease has been at number one for a long time. The major risk factor? Not your diet. It is *dissatisfaction*. In TCM, this is the wood element, controlled by the liver and the gallbladder. The wood feeds the fire (heart); when the wood is wet due to emotions such as disillusionment, frustration and sadness, the fire element becomes weak and cannot sustain itself.

The liver and gallbladder play an important role in the metabolism of cholesterol and fats. When cholesterol levels go haywire, it is not due to nutritional problems but due to emotional imbalances. The pharmaceutical industry earns billions with cholesterol-lowering drugs without ever coming close to addressing the real cause. The best remedy for the heart is letting go and accepting. In Japanese this is called *shoganai*. Accept what you cannot change – act upon what you can!

One of the landmark publications about heart disease and the emotions was the book *Type A Behavior and Your Heart* by Meyer Friedman, MD, and Ray H. Rosenman, MD, both cardiologists. They found type A personalities have a higher risk of fatal heart disease. Typical extreme type As are impatient, irritable, aggressive, fast-talking people prone to be workaholics. They are the typical hard-worker type (Level 1) and are into *competitive happiness*.

The good news is: this is not an inborn personality flaw; it's nothing but a learned pattern of behaviour, which can be changed. The most important characteristic of this personality is that it is easily roused to anger and impatience. The most important skill to learn is to change the pace and, instead of working hard, learn to work smart and be more intuitive. Not shoot from the hip but listen. Eat more slowly, wait patiently in lines or traffic, talk slower and really become interested in others.

The Enemy of Your Heart: Suppressed Anger

The key ingredient here is *hostility*. Hostility is not only the leading heart-disease risk, it is also associated with death from many other causes as well. This hostility is a basic lack of trust in human nature and motives. It is based on the self-fulfilling prophecy that people are more bad than good – they will judge you, cheat you and mistreat you. In the next chapter we will look at how beliefs always are self-fulfilling prophecies. A study done by Dr Williams and others at Duke University evaluated over 400 people for hostility and Type A behaviour. The subjects also underwent tests for arteriosclerotic plaques. The hostility levels were a much more accurate predicting factor for heart disease than other Type A behaviour patterns. Some 70 per cent with high hostility scores had arteriosclerotic plaques, compared to 50 per cent with low hostility scores. In other studies a six-fold higher incidence of heart disease was imminent in people with high hostility scores. So the key here is to learn to relax.

The best types of therapy for this personality type are meditation, Qigong, Tai Chi, yoga, walking in nature, listening to relaxing music, chanting and other types of relaxation. Yang conditions are balanced with yin therapy. I will introduce you to special acupressure points that will calm the yang-Wood energy when combined with specific affirmations.

The other positive news is that touch such as massage, hugging, stroking and social interactions are great stress-busters.

CANCER

Dr James J. Lynch, PhD, of the Center for Study of Human Psychophysiology at the University of Maryland's School of Medicine in Baltimore has discovered that people who live by themselves have much higher incidences of disease and premature death. Links to cancer and isolation have also been found. Cancer is another major killer. Dr Joan Borysenko, PhD, of Harvard Medical School is a psychologist and cell-biologist and is among a group of doctors looking at the link between personality and cancer. She has found in her research that cancer-prone people have had, in general, a poor relationship with their parents. Dr Richard B. Schekelle, PhD, professor of epidemiology at the University of Texas School of Public Health in Houston, has found that men who score highest on tests for depression have twice the rate of cancer as a control group. Depression has been shown to be associated with a weakened immune response. People with less anxiety and fear show less impaired immune response than their more stress-prone counterparts.

Other studies have found that a majority of cancer sufferers have lost a way to express themselves creatively. Other doctors have found that anger-suppression is also a significant risk factor. In cases of breast cancer it has been found that a large percentage of women having malignancies felt angry more often than women with benign tumours. Women with cancer were more apologetic about their anger, even when they felt they were right, while women with benign tumours tended to get angry and stay angry. Women with neither benign nor malignant tumours were more likely to blow up and then let go of it. They redirected their focus and energies toward more pleasant things.

LONGEVITY IS DIMINISHED BY UNRESOLVED EMOTIONS

Another area where emotions and attitude have a huge effect is longevity. People who are physically active will be prone to less depression and anxiety, and experience better mental efficiency, higher self-esteem, more restful sleep, more relaxation, spontaneity, enthusiasm and better self-acceptance (*Journal of Clinical Psychology* 1971; 27: 411-12). My belief is that physical exercise is one way to support the energy flow in the meridians.

Meridians are best compared to rivers of electricity flowing through the body. Unresolved emotions are like big stones in the river, causing resistance. By exercising we increase the force of the river and thus the stones are easier to overcome. Specific exercises for energy-flow, such as Qigong, Tai Chi, meditation and yoga, have an even greater effect on our emotional state.

Another finding is that smoking and other forms of addictions are never physical, always emotional. Smoking is one of the best ways to suppress the emotions. Nicotine addiction is easier to overcome with special acupressure techniques that remove the blockages in the meridians caused by years of emotional suppression. One of the things you want to work on is to get rid of all addictions in order to free yourself of blockages to emotional balance.

Emotional balance is very important to longevity. Research on ageing concludes that feeling connected with other people, having a purpose in life and also curiosity are all boons to longevity.

THE SKILL TO MASTER: LETTING GO OF THE PAST

My findings on people who stay healthy, even to a very old age, is that the most reliable factor they all have in common is the ability to let go of mishaps, loss and life's curve balls. If we can learn from these, we discover the first law of emotional balance: accepting what happens without losing sight of what you can do to make change happen. Helplessness and feeling like a victim are the surest ways to get your immune system into trouble. How you feel changes your energetic state and your biochemical/physiological state. In other words, if you are depressed, your immune system is depressed and will be overrun by invaders. Unresolved emotions will turn against you and cause damage to your system (organs and tissues). It's estimated by some researchers that 90 per cent of all physical problems have psychological roots. I believe this is no exaggeration. On the contrary, it may even be more than that. There's enough evidence available to show that virtually every disease is influenced for better or worse by our emotions. Once you know that there is a 97 per cent effective cure rate of chronic diseases as a result of practising a simple mind-body method such as Zhineng Qigong for just 30 to 50 days, then you may agree that the mind has a tremendous effect on our energy. That's one of the objectives of Qigong: to redirect our body's energy and harmonize all systems. One of the most common side-effects of practising Qigong is the happiness encountered in most practitioners. This newfound state of bliss is one of the reasons to continue practising.

THE MIND IS YOUR MOST POWERFUL HEALING TOOL

For me and many other researchers it is clear that the mind is the most powerful healing tool available to humanity. Through such techniques as acupressure, Qigong, meditation, self-hypnosis, bio-feedback, Reiki and therapeutic touch, we can flood the brain with positive healing images and messages that will be translated into biochemistry, the language of the body. Energy is the forming matrix for matter. If there are unresolved emotions, there will be disharmony. Disharmony will disrupt the cell's electrical fields and thus affect the integrity of the system, making us prone to disease. On the other hand, any form of dis-ease is a signal to look inside for the real cause. Even a common cold is a sign to look inward and check what is stressing you. Which emotions are unresolved?

Time to Journal

What is bothering you? What are you anxious, worried and fearful about? How is your self-esteem? Do you feel vulnerable, attacked, threatened? Where are your fears right now in your life? Are you focused on creating spiritual growth and discovering who you really are?

Every discomfort is turbulence. Turbulence is caused by unresolved emotions. If you do not act then you will re-experience the same or similar turbulence sooner or later. (I will show you how to get into action.)

Stress is not about external factors, it's about what you let those external factors do to your internal factors.

CHAPTER 2

TRIGGERS: REFLECTIONS OF OUR SHADOW WORLD

THE MIND CREATES ITS OWN ILLUSIONS

All the great teachers of our time tell us the same thing: 'We create our own reality.' For most of us, this is very hard to believe. If this is true, why do we create so much misery, war, poverty and suffering? In order to understand that everything that happens in our outer world is a reflection of what is happening in our inner world, we need to delve a little into the field of quantum physics.

ENERGY AND FIELDS

In Chapter 1 we spoke about energy and fields. Emotions, beliefs and other non-material qualities such as intuition, drive, motivation, creativity and wisdom originate in the dynamic chaos of our energetic body. This energetic field vibrates at a certain frequency and interacts with other energetic fields.

Let's go deeper into the consequences of this. It is known that matter consists of 99.999 per cent space and only 0.001 per cent atoms. What we see is an illusion created by the movements of these atoms. It's like a film: due to the speed of the frames per second, the movements on screen appear smooth and real.

The electromagnetic spectrum is vast. Visible light makes up less than a one-hundred billionth part of this spectrum. What we can see is nothing compared to what we cannot see. Even the things that we can see, we interpret differently due to the way we filter information based on our past experiences. Perception is nothing but our subjective distortion. That's why each individual will experience the same incident differently. If we were to rely exclusively on our five senses, we would have a very poor understanding of reality. Luckily, humans are wired with more than just these five senses, and by becoming aware of these and using them we can evolve to Level 2. At this level we start feeling resonances that are totally different from those at Level 1.

SUBTLE INTERACTIONS AND SELF-CREATED REALITIES

Each person, through his energy fields, interacts with the fields of other living beings and with stimuli from the environment. We can also be negatively affected by electromagnetic fields from electrical equipment. A fraction of the energetic information we are exposed to enters our energetic fields and we become aware of it through our senses, thoughts or intuition. The biggest part of the energetic fields that has an effect on us, however, remains hidden from our perception.

'Uninvited' input can come from other people as well. Even people with the best of intentions can affect us through their thoughts, worries and concerns. In her study of the human energy field, Dr Valerie Hunt recorded brain waves, galvanic skin responses, heart rate and blood-pressure changes and muscle contractions of patients while aura-readers observed changes in their energy fields. Dr Hunt discovered that changes occurred in the energy fields *before* they were measurable in any of the other bodily systems (*Townsend Letter for Doctors* 150: pp.124-26).

Let's move on to the concept of how we create our own reality. A good example is exam tension. This is a very common stress that has a clear cause: mild tension or anxiety is normal during an exam. It helps students improve their focus and pace. But when this stress is severe, students may experience negative thoughts or beliefs such as 'I will fail' or 'I can't remember anything.' These thoughts can often create physical symptoms such as fear, sleep loss, lack of appetite, loose stools, nausea, restlessness, frequent urination, headaches, aggression, irritability and giddiness. This can in turn have a severe impact on performance. For some, the fear will become real and they will indeed fail the exam and thus confirm their negative beliefs. In other words, fear can create precisely what we *don't* want.

Our thoughts, beliefs and perceptions affect every single cell in our body. Understanding the power of our emotions is the key to our health. Recurrent thoughts or attitudes, particularly, set the stage for health or illness. Triggers are stimuli that come from within or outside of us.

Let's look at how triggers affect our bodies. In the study of psychoneuroimmunology (PNI) the connection between mind–emotion–immune system is researched. The central nervous system and the immune system are linked in the following two ways.

1. Every Thought Is Translated into Biochemical Language

Research done by neurobiologist Candace Pert shows that emotionally-charged thoughts and memories cause the body to manufacture different neuropeptides (small protein-like molecules used by neurons to communicate with each other). Researchers at the Institute of Heart Math (Boulder, Colorado) found that positive emotions raise the body's levels of DHEA (a hormone that rejuvenates and fights stress) and IgA (an immune-protein), while negative emotions lower both. The neuropeptides have an effect not only on the brain but on all organs, glands, cells and tissues. Every thought we think and every emotion we feel is communicated to every cell in our bodies. Furthermore, the organs can store emotional information, too. This is becoming ever more evident now that organ transplants are more and more common.

Holographic Memory in Every Cell

Paul Pearsall's book *The Heart's Code* describes 73 cases of 'memory transplants' coinciding with heart transplants. In one case a murder case was solved as a result of a transplanted memory. One elderly woman started to crave the same foods her donor had done; another started speaking words from a language that had been the donor's native tongue. The list goes on and on. Pearsall suggests that cells communicate electromagnetically, and that memory can be stored in every cell.

In this way every cell becomes a hologram for the whole body. The concept that a heart-cell is just a cell no longer holds. We can now state that all organs and cells store emotional information.

2. The Autonomic Nervous System

The other way the central nervous system is linked to the immune system is through the autonomic nervous system.

The autonomic nervous system is divided into two parts: parasympathetic (PNS) and sympathetic (SNS). These are the yin and the yang of the nervous system. The PNS is the yin side and promotes growth, regeneration and assimilation. It will work best during relaxation and rest. It's the way we create a buffer that will help us through stressful times. The SNS is a reactive system that monitors external stimuli and adapts to these: noise, temperature, pain, etc. The SNS is part of our body's survival mechanism and can prepare us in an instant for intense muscular action. The PNS is inner-directed to the emotions and perceptions; the SNS has an outward focus. In modern life the SNS has become more dominant due to the fast pace of life, overload of information, work pressure, etc. For that reason tools to support the PNS have become essential. Again, here the most important ones are meditation, Tai Chi, Qigong and relaxation.

HOW PERCEPTIONS AFFECT OUR BIOLOGY

Let's suppose you are doing very well in your current job. Due to your excellent performance, your supervisor offers you a promotion, and now you manage all the people who once were your peers. Let's say your initial response is one of sheer excitement. You will get a 50 per cent increase in salary, a company car, extra bonuses, etc. You feel thrilled. Your brain will produce chemicals that correspond with this state, and all the cells will be excited. There will be a PNS response, increasing the parasympathetic activity in the body (and the levels of beta endorphins). This is good news and your buffer zone (your adaptability to stress) increases. After a while, other thoughts start creeping up: you realize that you are one of the youngest managers and have to supervise people old enough to be your parents. Now fear starts coming into play and you are worried about living up to the company's expectations. These fears will cause an SNS reaction and subsequent secretion of chemicals, such as norepinephrine, which communicates, chemically, the bad news to all cells. Your body goes into an alarm state and your adrenals are activated to produce a powerful hormone called *cortisol*. This is the so-called fight or flight response. The same message can trigger two opposite reactions in our bodies, based upon where we are with our focus at any given moment.

HOW OUR THOUGHTS CAN MAKE US ILL

Our bodies are governed by our energy systems. The two parts of our energetic body that we know most about are the meridians (energetic circulatory system) and the chakras (major energy centres). Also of major importance is the energy field that surrounds us. This is the electromagnetic field which allows us to know when someone behind us is looking at us. It's also the foundation of our intuition and so-called sixth sense (these forms of extrasensory perception become more active when we are at Level 2 of manifestation). This energy field also has a spiritual function, being a connection between the soul and the physical body.

Our energy patterns do not change. Our blueprint remains the same. When our energy system is out of balance, weak or damaged, problems will develop in our other systems, such as the digestive system, the endocrine system and the connective tissue.

What weakens or damages the energy-body?

TRIGGERS

Everything that happens to us has an effect: injury, illness, traumas, thoughts and beliefs. If we are already weakened by other challenges preceding a new stressor, the impact will be even greater.

So let's see how many triggers you recognize.

Thoughts Associated with Something You Hear

- Someone says something critical about your performance.

- Some people find their own voice on tape very unpleasant and unsettling.
- Certain music, sounds, voices can trigger acute reactions.
- Some people cannot sleep unless it's absolutely quiet. Others need soothing sounds to fall asleep.
- The voices of certain people may be a source of irritation.

Thoughts Associated with What You See

- Seeing your ex-wife or ex-husband with someone else.
- Some people are extremely upset by the sight of blood and violence.

Touch-triggers

- The body can have specific locations that carry negative memories.
- Certain ways of touching can set an inner alarm off.
- Lots of people are very sensitive about being touched, hugged or kissed.

Smell-triggers

- Smell can be pleasant or unpleasant, but besides that, smell can trigger specific responses in us.
- The smell of a perfume or eau de cologne can bring back memories from the past.

Taste-triggers

- Our taste buds also play a role in the triggering process. Whenever I taste porridge, I am reminded of a time when I was growing up and something unpleasant happened.

The important clue is that all unpleasant triggers are very significant signs of unresolved issues. The subconscious mind is reminding us to look at these issues. If we ignore these triggers, we are missing the chance to resolve important emotional issues in our lives.

Time to Journal

Write in your journal which triggers you recognize the most, and add as many more as you can think of.

OUR INNER PROCESSING

The next category of triggers is not related to our senses; they are linked to our own internal processes. We can wake up feeling terrible for no obvious reason. We can have mood swings, be depressed by the weather or after talking to someone. Here we also have the subconscious mind at work, trying to draw our attention to issues that we are not consciously aware of. By neglecting these opportunities for healing, we are continuing on the path that will lead to self-destruction or illness.

Other feelings can come up for no reason whatsoever, without any possible trigger. There is always a chance that we are tuned in or resonating with other people's energies or emotions. Other energies can have an impact on the rhythm, frequency, wavelength and electromagnetic charges of the energy waves that form our energetic body. This is called *resonance*. For anyone to pick up something from someone else there must be a similar energy structure in their system. In other words: the energy waves in your body can only change if they resonate with the energy waves of someone else.

TOXIC EMOTIONS CAUSE TRIGGERS

Triggers of any sort can only happen if there is a toxic emotion in your system. A toxic emotion is an unresolved emotion or a misinterpreted emotion that has not been released and is trapped in your internal energetic memory system. A given emotion does not release a specific chemical in your nervous system, however. It's the *meaning* or *interpretation* that we have given to that specific feeling that creates the biochemical reaction. This again will trigger disease and imbalances in your body.

Emotions are neither good nor bad; they are our guiding force. When we feel good (differentiate here between competitive, conditional and unconditional happy feelings), we are guided on a path to health and fulfilment. Unpleasant emotions are warning signs for us to take a closer look at our behaviour or perception. Triggers that cause unpleasant feelings should always be welcomed, as they are offering us a chance to change and get closer to unconditional happiness. Through our perceptions we can create our own health by paying attention to those things that bring us gratitude, joy, fun and a feeling of wellbeing. You may have no control over what happens in the world, but you have absolute control over how you deal with those events.

Each day, each moment in our lives offers us the opportunity of a new beginning, a new moment to let go of those things that no longer serve us. If we do not take this responsibility in our hands, we will buy into the disempowering belief that things happen *to* us and that we are a victim of circumstance. When you see yourself as a victim, then that's what you will be and your energetic body will respond accordingly. But if you free yourself from those disempowering beliefs and feelings by not fighting them, but by accepting them without judging, you take the first step toward freeing yourself from the past. Freedom from the past means free-flowing energy, no more blockages caused by memories or thoughts. How you will get there is the subject of this book; in Part II, we will focus on more practical tools.

It is clear that triggers are the best opportunity for growth; so let me repeat myself and bring this closer to home. The word I will use for triggers will be *turbulence*. You are in a traffic jam, late for an important meeting and your mobile phone's battery is dead. How do you feel? If you feel upset, frustrated, angry, anxious or anything besides *shoganai* (acceptance of what you cannot change and getting on with your life), or bliss (happiness despite the unpleasant situation), you are being triggered and need to take a serious look at yourself. Looking at it from a Level 1 consciousness, you are right to feel frustrated.

SHOGANAI
When we are at Level 2 of consciousness, we take responsibility for this situation and connect with our intuition.

We need to check the following:

- Is there a reason why this meeting may not be good for me now?
- What are the consequences if this turns out to be a positive meeting?
- What will I have to give up because of this success?
- What am I afraid of losing? Am I ready for this level of success?
- Do I have any doubts or bad feelings about this?

Go as deep as you can. Focus on your inner knowing by detaching from the outcome and meditating. Once you create silence and feel at ease, you will see what comes up from inside of you, from the place that knows everything.

- Which signs have I neglected that could have prevented this from happening?
- What led to this series of events creating this situation?
- What did I overlook?
- What other precautions should I have taken?
- What can I do now (for example: get off the motorway and to a public phone if possible)?
- Why would I have created this? What are the benefits (perhaps having more time to prepare)?

Of course we cannot foresee everything; but you will be surprised how much you can come up with if you really give this a try. Everything in our lives happens for a reason, and the outcome in the long run is *always* for our own good.

HIGHER LEVELS OF AWARENESS

When we look at the events from a Level 3 consciousness – the level of effortlessness – we understand that this is the best of all circumstances, because we have created it. We know there is an intention behind it, this is our intent and we already know what it is. So, whenever we are in the midst of turbulence, we first need to go to that state: the state of effortlessness. This is the state of trust in the divine intent connecting with our own intent and aligning the two. It is the state of acceptance, forgiveness and letting go. It is the path of least resistance, not because we want to avoid work, but because we know that we get more done when we allow the universe to do its work. If we experience situations that trigger emotions or turbulence in ourselves, we immediately know that it has nothing to do with the external stimuli, but everything to do with some unresolved issue in ourselves. By not resisting or fighting the turbulence, but by loving it, we transform it.

The well-known therapist Gay Hendricks has noted that any area of pain, blame or shame in our lives is there because we have not loved that part of ourselves enough. The best way to get an 'unpleasant' feeling such as guilt or shame to go away is simply by loving yourself for having it. By accepting these feelings or thoughts effortlessly and not spending energy judging them, and moving on, you literally free yourself to be creative again. The energy circulates freely again and the effect of the turbulence is gone.

The third level of consciousness also makes possible the emergence of a new paradigm. There is now, despite powerful countervailing trends, a deep pattern-shift occurring in global values – a shift toward a more conscious living system perspective. The condition of the world mirrors our collective consciousness. More and more people are experiencing themselves as masters of their environment, as active creators in a pre-existing world. Consciousness becomes more and more a causal reality. This action of consciousness at all levels of reality results in quantum phenomena that can be scientifically validated at all strata of science. That is as long as science is not pursuing the natural motivation of the human brain, which is an effort after 'meaning', rather than an effort after 'truth'.

In conclusion, all turbulence (no matter what we call it: triggers, stress, distress, injury, accidents, coincidence, bad luck, etc.) is a reflection of our own consciousness and happens with a specific intention. Although the intention is always good, our awareness of it can belie this.

CHAPTER 3

SELF-SABOTAGE

THE PAST IS A DEDICATED TEACHER

In the first chapter we looked at the effects of emotions as energetic phenomena that can turn against our internal balance and contribute to chronic disease. In the second chapter we considered the concept that what we experience in our day-to-day reality is an expression of inner turmoil. When we take this one step further to the third level of consciousness, we understand that we've created our circumstances with a certain intention. When we look back in time and evaluate our lives, we will see many times where our feelings got in the way and prevented us from behaving the way we really wanted to. Our emotions determine, to a great extent, our responses. We sometimes blow up because of little things; maybe you were tired after a hard day at work. After eight hours of being Mr Nice Guy, we let our guard down and don't have the patience we should have for our loved ones. The good news is that people are like oranges: what's inside comes out when you squeeze them. If there is a lot of bitterness or anger inside, the juice will be bitter. The best news is that with diligent practice of some simple techniques, we can replace the bitterness with sweetness and pleasure. So, even when we are physically tired, we can still evolve to show our love and kindness to our loved ones or anyone else. Our inability to cope emotionally comes basically from self-rejection (we will get into this more later on); let us first have a look at how the juice that's inside comes out.

Disempowering Feelings

Here the response to stressful events is with emotions such as helplessness, despair, frustration, anger, jealousy, feelings of inadequacy, shame or guilt and so on. These feelings can be triggered by a phone call, letter or email from someone who criticizes us, something our spouse does that we don't like, or a misbehaving pet. Anything can provoke the bitter juice from the orange.

Self-defeating Coping Behaviour
Many people do not know how to deal with certain emotions once they feel them. They may flee by withdrawing, abusing mind-altering substances (such as alcohol, medication and drugs) or mood-altering substances (such as foods, cigarettes). They may also respond in an overly aggressive way, shouting or throwing tantrums. Alternatively, they may go to complete indifference and external calmness.

Negative Beliefs
Others may have the tendency to believe it's 'wrong' to have certain emotions or feelings, such as anger, frustration and desire. When they experience these emotions, they feel extreme shame or guilt.

Self-destructive Behaviour
Some respond to situations they can't handle emotionally by doing things that are very dangerous. There is a subconscious death wish and they subconsciously welcome injuries and the attention they get as a result.

The foundation of all these ways of responding to external stimuli is based on how we see ourselves. Self-esteem is essential for emotional survival; without sufficient self-worth, life is a painful experience and we miss out a lot that is fulfilling and gratifying. We are different from animals in that we have the capacity to create and value ourselves accordingly. The irony is that we create an image of ourselves and then judge this image. Most people do not fully like the image they've created; any rejection of this image is self-rejection and the major cause of most of our problems. This is the biggest challenge of being human, because when we reject our image or parts of ourselves, we are weakening and destroying the psychological foundation that keeps us alive. We cause our own inner noise or turbulence. We reject and judge ourselves constantly and inflict unnecessary pain. This is a downward spiral that will lead eventually to avoiding anything that may worsen the pain of self-rejection. We create all sorts of defence mechanisms and avoid confrontation. The worst part is that we lose our objectivity and intuition. We filter everything based on whether a given thing is something to avoid, deny, suppress, blame or criticize. We limit our ability for intimacy, expressing our feelings, hearing criticism and asking for help or solving our conflicts. The end result is that we have no emotional choice – we become victims of our own shadows – and are emotional hostages with limited capacity to respond. The results are almost always the same:

- disempowering feelings
- self-defeating behaviour
- negative beliefs
- self-destructive behaviour

Time to Journal

Before we continue, take a moment of silence and reflect on what you've read so far. Do you recognize anything that you experience yourself? If you do, how would you like to change that? What do you feel is holding you back from making that change? What resource would you need in order to make that change? What can you do to have more access to that resource?

The biggest illusions that we need to overcome are:

1. External factors create stress in us.
2. Asking for help when we are stressed (or ill).

Once you see through these illusions you are already halfway to emotional balance. If we are, ourselves, the cause of our internal mayhem, then we had better take control of the command centre and learn how to steer clear of the rocky road. The only help we need from outside is a course on

24

how to take control of our own lives, and how to create for ourselves a supportive network. The essence is that everything that is important comes from within. This is the first clue to inner harmony. We need to accept ourselves, accept that life is difficult, that there will be roadblocks, that we will make a lot of mistakes and that many people will believe that we are the source of their misery.

Please read this section again at least two times and do not continue until you grasp it completely.

Journal your most important insights for deeper reflection.

LOVE THE FACT THAT NOT EVERYONE WILL LIKE YOU

There will be people who do not like you – and that should be OK. We cannot please everyone. It is important to grasp that, due to our childhood survival training, most of us learned some or all of the following:

1. *Your parents are the boss*; their commands should be followed under all circumstances, unless you can get away with it.
2. *They are always right*, because they know better and are clairvoyant (they can see your future).
3. *Although you are absolutely sure you are right*, rule 2 is still in force.
4. You will love them unconditionally because they created you, give you food and shelter and get you toys (which is *conditional love*).
5. You must suppress all emotions that could be interpreted as you not loving them or as you disagreeing with them.
6. Behaving in a socially acceptable manner helps you to exert tremendous power over how the boss feels. With certain behaviour you can make them feel bad, unhappy or the opposite: happy and blissful. *You are responsible for how they feel*.

7. If you do not behave in an acceptable and favourable manner, you are bad and not loveable. You will be rejected and possibly deserted.

8. Most of your real emotions are not acceptable; they will have a negative impact on your boss.

9. The boss does not have to keep his/her promises, but you have to keep yours under all circumstances.

10. The boss can do bad things to their health and wellbeing, because they are older and 'wiser'. You should refrain from these things until you are old enough to destroy yourself.

These are the rules I remember still from 45 years ago when I underwent the survival training that was meant to help me cope with life. At that time these were useful. If we do not let go of this outdated model of reality, however, we make ourselves prone to mental illness.

Psychiatrists refer to clinging to an outdated concept of reality as *transference*. Transference is the way we perceive and respond to external stimuli, which is developed in our childhood and which in childhood was appropriate survival behaviour but which is then inappropriately transferred into our adult reality.

When we are children, our parents are the world. They are representatives of our future values, the world as we see it. We assume that the way our parents do things is **The Way**. The truth is that if you discover, for instance, that you cannot trust your parents, this will be translated as: 'You cannot trust people.' The length and quality of the time that our parents devote to us forms the basis for our self-love and self-esteem. All children are terrified of abandonment, because for the child abandonment is the equivalent of death. If we do not get a base of security and reassurance, the world will be an unsafe place to be.

One of the big problems that we may have is a parent who is overly protective. They often want to help so much that they don't give us the chance to develop problem-solving skills. Later in life we will expect others to solve our problems and we will not take responsibility for ourselves.

Another area that may be lacking is discipline. Discipline is the greatest and most important factor in success but also in spiritual growth. Most people shy away from spiritual growth because they expect it demands too much discipline. In Dr M. Scott Peck's book *The Road Less Traveled*, he wrote the following:

Let us teach ourselves and our children the necessity for suffering and the value thereof, the need to face problems directly and to experience the pain involved. I have stated that discipline is the basic set of tools we require to solve life's problems. It will become clear that these tools are techniques of suffering, means by which we experience the pain or problems in such a way as to work them through and solve them successfully, learning and growing in the process. When we teach ourselves and our children discipline, we are teaching them and ourselves how to suffer and also how to grow.

Dr Peck mentions four tools of discipline:

1. delaying of gratification
2. acceptance of responsibility
3. dedication to truth
4. the art of balancing.

As we can see, most inner turmoil comes from:

1. wanting instant gratification
2. avoiding our responsibility
3. being untruthful to ourselves and others
4. not being able to handle the curve balls that life keeps throwing at us.

Whenever we face inner turbulence, we must be able to stay connected with ourselves.

The worst we can do is:

- Go back to our childhood survival rules.
- Adopt the parent's role by criticizing and rejecting our behaviour/performance.
- Refrain from nurturing and loving ourselves.

SELF-REJECTION IS THE CAUSE

After 30 years of dealing with sick people, my conclusion is the following: all inner turbulence (emotional stress) comes from self-rejection.

Where does this self-rejection come from? We all have a so-called Inner Judge, which we normally hear as a voice in our head. This Inner Judge is the by-product of our upbringing. We have been conditioned and trained for survival by our caretakers teaching us which behaviours are wrong, bad, dangerous, annoying, loveable, acceptable and good. If we did not live up to their expectations we were punished one way or another. All of us will have emotional residues from this training. These are conscious (and also subconscious) memories of all the times we felt bad or rejected. We also had an almost impossible task to differentiate between behaviour and identity. When we were disciplined or corrected often, we believed that we as a person were flawed and that we were hopeless and bad. These are the unavoidable subtle traumas that have a tremendous effect on our self-esteem. This experience is the foundation of the Inner Judge, who will replace our parents and will feed on the unpleasant feelings associated with the part of our identity or behaviour that we consider not OK. There is a *subconscious* program in you that wants you to believe that you are a bad person as soon as someone does not agree with you or is upset or does not like you, or when you make a mistake or do not finish a task. The Inner Judge confirms some negative belief you already have of yourself.

There are six main factors that will determine how strongly you will reject yourself:

1. **The degree to which your parents failed to make a distinction between your identity and your behaviour**

   Most of us do not learn that there is a huge difference between what we do (behaviour) and who we are (identity). Parents should always reinforce and show their love for our identity, and their disapproval of certain behaviours. This is best done with a technique called 'sandwich feedback':

   - First layer: tell the child what he is doing right.
   - Second layer: tell him what needs improvement and how you would like to see that improvement.
   - Third layer: thank him for his willingness to listen and cooperate, and state how proud you are of him.

   Unfortunately most parents are not aware of this technique, with the result that later in life our Inner Judge will criticize both our behaviour and identity, and tell us that we are no good and that we will always fail.

2. **The degree to which issues are mislabelled as moral when they are about personal needs and/or safety**

   Let's say that a child prefers certain clothes because all her friends have them, and you lecture her on the lower social class of her friends. Or when addressing performance in school, a father tells his son how he makes him feel ashamed or that the son is so ungrateful for all the sacrifices he makes to send him to school. Whenever parents make their children feel morally wrong because of failure to perform, poor judgement or personal preferences, this will lead to self-worth problems.

3. **The frequency of negative messages**

   The average 16-year-old has heard around 180,000 times what she is not good at, what she should not do, why she doesn't deserve something, how badly she behaves, and other negative messages. 'What's wrong with you?' 'Can't you ever get anything right?' 'Are you stupid?'

Sooner or later these messages will sink in and become future weapons for her Inner Judge.

4. **The consistency of discipline (rules)**

   Children will constantly challenge their parents to check their consistency on the rules. If there is randomness and/or inconsistencies, as when the parents are tired, rules can go by the wayside. Only one conclusion can be reached: that you are punished, not for something you do, but for who you are. Guilt is often associated with inconsistency around enforcing rules.

5. **Rejection by one's parents**

   When a parent rejects a child by withdrawing or ignoring him or being and staying very angry about something, a great deal of damage to the self-esteem can be done. This, for the child, confirms that he is not worthwhile or loveable.

6. **Verbal abuse and verbal rejection**

   When parents verbally abuse their children and tell them repeatedly that they are worthless and not loveable, this is the worst damage that one can imagine together with physical and sexual abuse. This will leave deep emotional scars that will influence future self-esteem levels tremendously.

These are the most important reasons we reject ourselves and often become our own worst enemies and critics. They're also the reasons why a lot of people stay stuck at the first level of consciousness. No matter how hard they work to prove themselves, deep inside there will be all these demons that will create havoc and prevent inner peace.

We all have certain basic needs which, when not addressed or dealt with properly, can turn against us and cause us inner turmoil.

We all want to feel:

- secure and free of fear
- accepted by others (preferably loved by others)

- competent and adequate
- self-worth and self-sufficient in most situations.

When we have adequate self-esteem, we will have totally different approaches and strategies than when we lack self-esteem.

When we can handle situations from a place of inner strength, we are able to:

- Confront our fears and find solutions.
- Accept that not everyone will like us or accept us.
- Accept that we cannot be competent in all areas of life, and that, if we want something badly enough, we will pursue it and work around the roadblocks.
- Cope with interpersonal conflicts and not avoid them.
- Accept that we are not perfect and will make mistakes.

When we are low on self-esteem, everything becomes different. Life is much more difficult to handle and often we look for hide-outs and escape. We cope with anxiety and conflicts by avoiding the situation that causes these feelings of inadequacy. Your Inner Judge offers help with this. The big paradox is that, despite the harshness and the negativity of the Inner Judge, he does make you feel better. Your belief that you are worthless will be confirmed; people don't love you, and you cannot trust anyone. Now you can relax because there is no need to be anxious; you will feel less incompetent, less vulnerable. The best cop-out is to buy into the following statements: 'There is nothing I can do about it,' 'I am the way I am,' 'If I had been brought up differently, everything would have been different!'

The reason this issue is so important has to do with the impact our thoughts and feelings have on our energetic body. Wherever thought goes, energy and life-force follow. Most people are aware of energy being lost in the form of emotional ties and binding with other human beings and even pets. Most of us are not aware of how much life energy we spent on past incidents, regrets, old beliefs (often not even our own beliefs) and losses. Our thoughts of each moment indicate where our energy is flowing. When thoughts contain negative messages, underlying fear, lack of self-esteem, anxiety, worries and hostility, energy is being lost or blocked in the body. When we are more focused on positive messages or images, or do not resist what we cannot change and let go of old grievances and insults, the energy will circulate to the areas that were previously blocked, and healing can take place.

In whatever way we use our life energy, whether we utilize it to focus on anger and frustration, or on joy and harmony, it will manifest in our biology. Prolonged disharmony or weakness in our energy field will lead to physical malfunction and illness.

THE MORPHOGENETIC FIELD OF CONSCIOUSNESS

Often, our thinking is random: thoughts come and go. Our thoughts are, however, also projected outside of us into the connecting field known as the *morphogenetic field*. This is an electromagnetic field that engulfs the world and connects each one of us directly with each other. Other people can pick up on our messages and also our intention. This is where the non-physical senses such as intuition and clairvoyance come into play. All of us have non-physical senses and extraordinary capabilities; most of us are unaware of this, yet we still react to the unheard, unseen and non-verbal messages of others. Everyone is projecting their thoughts and feelings into the morphogenetic field; there are no exceptions. When we connect a feeling and a thought, we get a judgement. Every judgement leads to an energetic block in our bodies. Every time we judge ourselves, we create energetic blocks in our meridian system. Every time we judge someone else, we also create energetic blocks in our own body.

Suppose you are upset with someone. Every time you see this person or think of this person, hear his name or any other possible association, the feeling of being upset will be there as well and create energy blocks in your system. The more we judge, the more we become hostage to our feelings and the more energy will be sapped from our meridian systems. This will cause rigidity and stiffness in our bodies. This will eventually lead to sickness and disease.

Judging Anything or Anybody Is Robbing Yourself of Life-force!

There is a difference between a judgement and an opinion. An opinion is not emotionally charged and is neutral. We can change opinions quite easily when we get new data or information. It's OK to have opinions, but as soon as you become attached to your opinion this will eat up energy. The key is to be non-attached and neutral.

The best way to deal with negative emotions is to focus on the feeling and not on the label or judgement of the feeling. What do we feel? Where do we feel it? How intense is this feeling? It is not even important to find the cause; the obvious cause is never the cause. It's a trigger that sets off alarm bells due to old memories. Accept the feeling, even if it's uncomfortable.

Suppose you have a negative thought about yourself and consequently you feel bad. You localize this as a heavy feeling in your stomach area. Then you completely accept this feeling and just be with it – thank your body for being such a perfect machine and warning you of this energy block in your system. The affirmation that I've found to be most powerful is: 'I love and accept myself with this feeling.' Send loving thoughts to the area in distress and visualize energy flowing freely through this area. Later on we will go deeper into the techniques that will assist you in speeding up this process.

The basis is simply accepting and loving ourselves, just the way we are. We don't have to change anything; we just need to connect with the love we already have inside of us. By not accepting ourselves unconditionally the way we are, we are rejecting ourselves or part of ourselves. The commandment 'Love thy neighbour as thyself' is based on the premise of loving ourselves first and unconditionally. Whenever we do not accept another person just the way he or she is, we are inflicting damage to ourselves. Accepting others does not mean agreeing with them or giving up our rights. It means accepting them the way they are without judgement, even when they do unpleasant things. The underlying energetic law is: *every person we reject is a reflection of a part of ourselves that we reject.*

In the end there is no difference between you and the other. We have created this moment in time and space and there is always something to be learned when we block our energies. Another way to look at it is to ask the question, 'How can I deal with this person or situation without losing energy?' Only when I accept others and every situation unconditionally, do I accept myself. Each and every incident, trauma, accident, situation, person is a part of my own creation, and thus I can accept and love it 100 per cent. In the beginning this can cost some energy, but it will become the path of least resistance. The path of least resistance leads to inner harmony, less loss of energy and unconditional loving of the self and others. Getting there will require dedication.

CHAPTER 4

KARMA AND EMOTIONS

WE ARE EMOTIONAL HOSTAGES TO OURSELVES

To experience life as beauty and goodness, without becoming enslaved to it, while being of service to others and remaining truthful to oneself – this sums up the basics of the law of karma.

For most people karma is linked to the philosophy of reincarnation. We will look into that in Chapter 7 and elaborate on it, but for this chapter we will focus on what karma is and how it relates to our emotions, and how this knowledge can change the entire course of our lives. This knowledge of karma will help us to make the optimum choices in our lives and help us turn painful memories and situations into opportunities for spiritual growth.

In order to understand fully what the law of cause and effect (karma) means, we need to look at life, not as a series of random events and incidents, but as part of a global network of interrelated souls, free to choose. There are no victims, no abusers, no victors nor losers; there is no such thing as bad luck, good luck, coincidence or destiny. There is no chaos. On the contrary, there is an orderly, coherent system governed by certain laws. All is predictable when all the factors are known. There is a predictable connection between our choices and the consequences.

The truth is that we are in control but often have given up our power and have become enslaved by our desires and needs. Once you accept that you do have control but have relinquished it, you will do what it takes to get back behind the steering wheel, won't you? The question is, how do you find your path through life? How are you guided? That's the difference between Level 1 of consciousness and the other levels.

Level 1: You Are Guided by Circumstances

Things happen to you; you can be lucky or have bad luck. Your approach to life is 'hit or miss'; this is caused by a lack of awareness or passivity and ultimately is self-denial. It's denial of your capacity and spirit. Life is like Russian roulette!

Level 2: You Trust Your Intuition and Follow What Feels Right

You start creating more synchronicity in your life and you accept that there are ups and downs. You start connecting and communicating with your guides, angels or Higher Self. You start understanding the signs and language of the universe.

Level 3: You Trust that You and the Universe Are One

What happens in your life is the reflection of your intentions. You choose to be pure and clear in your intent. There are no ups and downs, there is only now. In the now you are constantly letting go of the past.

WHAT EXACTLY IS THE LAW OF KARMA?

Let's understand what the law of karma means: there are two basic choices. Either we choose the bliss of ignorance or we choose to be aware of the fact that every action has its consequences. The latter means knowing we have to seize every opportunity to choose the very best for our lives. The law of karma means that you are always choosing; if you refuse to make a choice, your past will make that choice for you, because your old intent still stands.

By changing our original intent of childhood – which was, by the way, the subconscious programming of survival – we can evolve to a next level of being. Karma boils down to actions and our past experiences. Make a mental note here: *all actions generate memory.* This same memory will create a new desire to fulfil whatever was not resolved in the past. This desire that we are manifesting will drive us to action, which leads us to karma.

We can see what happens if we do not deal with our emotions: we become trapped in a vicious cycle that keeps reinforcing itself.

The circumstances will vary, but the underlying pattern will be the same. By understanding and accepting this law, we gain greater endurance and flexibility to get through the difficulties of life.

GET CONTROL OF WHAT IS CONTROLLABLE: SOLVING YOUR CONFLICTS

A dentist friend of mine is famous for being one of the few pain-free dentists in the country. People flock from everywhere to come and see him. In his office he has a button on the dentist's chair which you can hold on to during treatment. Whenever you feel the slightest discomfort, you can push the button and he will respond to your pain. He has the fewest requests for painkillers than any other dentist. The truth is that people very seldom make use of the button. The reason behind this is that, by having access to the button, people feel they have control. They are not helpless and, because of that, the biggest pain-inducer of all, anxiety, disappears.

It's the same with karma: when we take control it's much easier to deal with the difficulties that we create for ourselves. The main thing we need to accept is that nothing happens to us without our soul's consent and cooperation. Therefore, all of our reality is the product of our choices.

The beauty is that, even in our most difficult moments, there is the opportunity for maximum growth. The laws of the universe are no secret to us: they are as real as the law of gravity, and we are fully capable of making them work as we already understand them on a subconscious level. Our feelings are our inbuilt detectors of these universal laws. In the universe there is ultimate orderliness and harmony; as soon as we consciously tap into that, we can feel it. By tuning in to this feeling we can discern when we are doing something that disturbs this harmony. In other words, the law of karma aligns us with the ubiquitous harmony of the universe.

To understand the law of karma fully, we need to know that every thought, every desire that we feel, every emotion that we suppress will change our vibrational rate. We can use this to our advantage, as we can change our vibrational rate to attract what we want. We can learn how to do this through the techniques explained in this book.

As we get more insights into how this functions, we also make leaps of awareness and can transcend higher in the levels of consciousness. We have to develop in order to become 'multi-sensorial'. The five senses perceive only the physical, material world. This results in two opposite reactions at Level 1. Here we find the 'achievers', who would rather die than give up their dreams, and the people on 'cruise-control' – these are the masses, the majority. They accept their fate, and most will work at an unsatisfying job until they can retire and slowly deteriorate. Most of them are not happy at all and are very envious and critical of the 'achievers'. Often they are anti-capitalism, because they cannot compete. At this level, whoever accumulates the most wealth before death wins. This is also the level of the so-called rat-race.

Then we have the 'quietists'. They have given up and derive their quietude by accepting life as it is. They don't struggle anymore, and actually once they stop trying to achieve their dreams, they do find a sense of inner calm. The difference between these people and the 'cruise-controllers' is that they do not experience feelings of hostility.

In terms of karma, our choices and the actions they engender are our tools for evolving in consciousness. Each and every moment we choose the intentions that will give our experiences meaning. When we make choices based on our alignment with our higher consciousness, we can let go of many of the Level 1, primitive driving forces such as greed, security, fear, anger, revenge, shame, loneliness and our desire for external fulfilment. A multi-sensorial person is open to insights, intuition, sixth sense and other subtle feelings, signs and signals. This person will make choices based on love, compassion and wisdom, and will let go of negativity and being judgemental.

It is very obvious and it has been said many, many times: we have to become conscious of our choices. Any influence that limits our choices is our enemy.

To sum up: behind every incident, action, thought, feeling, need or desire is an intention. This intention comes from an original cause: unfinished business. When we act consciously, we can break this karmic cycle and create more space for positive, creative, loving energy and more effortlessness in our lives.

Once we incorporate the law of karma into our lives and we start to understand that all the people in our microcosm and all the events that take place are orchestrated by our collective superior consciousness, so all involved can evolve at their own pace and in their comfort zone.

The spiritual path is a series of choices you make that always carries the promise of greater harmony within itself. As with everything, at the beginning it takes practice and hard work. The only way to achieve effortlessness is through the discipline of following the path of least resistance; this can take a lot of practice in deconditioning and deprogramming ourselves from the beliefs of Level 1.

THE ULTIMATE DELAYED GRATIFICATION IS HEAVEN

We will face many crossroads where instant gratification will point us in the direction of dishonesty, selfishness or any other human vice. Often, the 'best' choices are the hard choices that require discipline, self-sacrifice and being of service to others. It is also the path of non-attachment and defencelessness. It is the path of allowing things to flow freely in our lives without the desire to hold on to things at any cost. The universal energy is the greatest source of energy; for it to flow through us, we need to liberate ourselves from our negative memories of the past, which block our energy flow. Any interference with the flow of this energy will reduce our affluence at Levels 2 and 3 of consciousness.

One of the sure ways to block the free flow of energy is to try to hold on to what we think we need: possessions, relationships, careers and people. This will also close the circle around us and block the influx of new things and people into our lives. The difference between having and holding is heaven. Whenever there is holding on to something, there is attachment.

Here is a simple rule: anything you cannot bring with you when you transcend out of the physical realm is not worth holding on to; it will only block the free flow of energy into your life. The most difficult paradox to understand is how this functions when you are in a relationship. You can have total devotion and commitment to the relationship, and trust your partner fully and completely, and yet not be attached at all. The relationship continues due to the moment-by-moment renewal of your commitment to that relationship. This also will be a choice you make on a continuous basis.

The main reason we want to hold on to things is that we do not trust that the universe will provide. Again, this mistrust is based on our past emotional reality; in this way we unknowingly create exactly what we wanted to prevent in the first place. We also believe that we know our needs better than the universe. On Levels 2 and 3 of consciousness we realize that by sharing our abundance and serving others, we will always be connected with the infinite source of energy available to us all the time.

To master the law of universal abundance, we have to let go of our limiting beliefs and any perceived shortage. At Level 3 we finally recognize that abundance is the natural state of being, and we release all attachments to material abundance and we can let it really flow freely into our lives.

HARMONY IS THE GOAL OF THE UNIVERSE

The law of karma is not an arbitrary code of behaviour or goodness in the universe; it is the way to maintain harmony within the universe. Here is the best part of all: any thought, action, belief or desire that is in resonance with the harmony of the universe will multiply into more harmony and love. Imagine three tuning forks: one is a huge tuning fork vibrating at a specific harmonious frequency; this attracts other people tuned in to the same type of frequency. Then there is another huge tuning fork that vibrates at a disharmonious frequency. The third one is our own tuning fork; you have a choice between harmonious and dissonant frequencies. Whatever you choose, it will be reinforced by one of the two bigger tuning forks and you will get back what you send out.

In summary: every action, thought, desire or feeling that is not in harmony with the goodness of the universe will come back to us sooner or later to give us a chance to get back in line with the universal harmony. So, actually karma is the best thing that can happen to you. It allows you to make a new choice again. The other good news is that there is no judge or God keeping Him- or Herself busy evaluating our actions and keeping a record.

The biggest limitation we face is trying to define a phenomenon of which we are an interactive part. Every observation is limited by the limitations of the observer. How can you measure with only five senses something that stretches infinitely beyond those senses? The law of karma is not about punishment; on the contrary, it is the law of mercy and love and is an expression of the interconnectedness between the universal intelligence and us. It is the law of communion and oneness, and the expression of the ultimate nature of goodness. Therefore, when we speak of karma we should differentiate between positive and negative karma.

What else is there to know about karma that may affect our lives? The more we understand, the better. It is important to realize that knowledge that does not lead to insights and better choices is also 'bad' karma. If you know that smoking cigarettes is bad for your health and you choose to continue smoking, that is 'bad' or 'negative' karma. If you choose to stop smoking because it is bad for you and others, you are building up 'good' karma. We need to become karma-recognition experts, one of the toughest skills to develop. This is the ability to trace specific causes and their effects; as a result, we will be better able to make choices that will bring 'good' karma to us. It will also allow us to accept more easily the consequences of past karma. The law of karma is not as simple as it seems; it is straightforward in principle, but very complex in its ramifications.

EMPOWERING BELIEFS

If we fully want to understand all of karma's complexity, we need to take into account the philosophy of reincarnation. If we put that into the equation, much more makes sense. Whether we believe in it or not does not change what is. Acceptance of reincarnation will help us only to understand better what we are possibly looking at. The second thing that is helpful is the belief that there is no such thing as an accident or random event, and nothing that occurs is anyone's fault or mistake. We all are part of a global conspiracy and we, on a certain level, have chosen to participate in this dance of life. Actually, we are enthusiastic volunteers who have agreed to the events that are happening right now. We can choose to step out at any given time, but to do so we need to be able to tune in and open up to the universal language. Some of the challenges we have right now come from childhood experiences, others are from previous lives.

The third empowering belief is that, whatever the challenge, we are up to the task. We are never in this alone; we are in this together and we can support each other. For those who have doubts about the law of karma and reincarnation, ask yourself the following question: 'What do I have to lose by accepting this as a possibility?' If you really think about it, the answer is nothing.

There is no way you can hurt yourself more than you may be doing right now. If the law does exist, you gain tremendous benefit by making use of it. If it does not, you can only become a better person for trying. Not accepting the law of karma simply means that there is no purpose, there is a random sequence of events over which you have no control whatsoever and you are powerless. You can also decide to test the validity of this law for at least a year. At least you will know that you have given yourself the opportunity to reclaim your creative power and have a big chance of improving the quality of your life. If we can agree on this, we can analyze the law of karma further and see what we can learn from the sages, who have a long tradition of studying it. Remember, *all news is good news* and we can only gain from knowledge if we act upon it.

The really good news about the law of karma is that, despite the fact that there are multitudinous ways it can express itself in our day-to-day lives, there are just a few basic categories that we need to grasp to know how it interacts with our choices.

First, the Sanskrit word *karma* means 'action'. I prefer the word 'choice'. Karma is about the choices we make and all the consequences of those choices.

THE FIRST LAW OF KARMA: THE LAW OF CONSERVATION

The law of conservation of mass and energy tells us that energy is never consumed but will only change form, and the total energy in any given physical system cannot be increased or diminished. This can also be called the law of continuation. It takes eight minutes for sunlight to reach us from its source. What we see as sunlight is an action that took place eight minutes ago. With the faraway stars this phenomenon is even more dramatic: what we see in the night sky can be information that is thousands of years old. This information travels on forever in time and space. The same concept, converted to our personal lives, suggests that there is a tendency for the effect of our choices or past actions to continue from lifetime to lifetime.

Most people believe that our participation is confined to just one life. After this life, all is finished. You come with a blank soul and leave with nothing else than the life experiences you've had. In Chapter 7 I will discuss with you why this is never true, and why we all come into this realm with a whole set of impurities in our system which have nothing to do with reincarnation or religion but are pure scientific facts. The multi-sensorial person is open to the possibility of repeated incarnations as a way to explain many mysteries of life, and knows that the spirit is the part of us that is immortal. The spirit is not limited to time or space. It experiences all incarnations at once. One change affects past, future and present, simultaneously.

I have seen this in practice over a thousand times. When a patient who has previously felt that he has been badly hurt by another person (for example, a parent) forgives that person from his heart, an immediate change can be observed. The memory of the event is instantaneously altered (the past); the future changes at the same time as the present. The person's physiology changes; even his biochemistry changes.

Change can happen in the blink of an eye. Often the other people involved also change. Our personality and physical body are tools through which the spirit evolves. Every aspect of the personality and physical body is adapted to suit the purpose of the spirit. By letting go of fear and all related limiting emotions, karma is changed immediately; each time we let go of one of our fears, we stop the projection of that into the future, back to the past and in the now, and we release one emotional hostage. The spirit is not time-bound, so the future and the past are not fixed. The goal is to let go of as much negativity (projected fear) as possible to get closer to our original blueprint of unconditional love. The good news about the karmic law of conservation is that no effort or intention is ever lost. Whatever you've gained in this life, emotionally and spiritually, you will bring with you into the next or into eternity. The energy and dedication we put into our efforts will determine the future effect of our labours. That is why it is important to discipline ourselves to continue with our spiritual practice, as we will reap the benefits sooner or later.

The downside of this karmic law is that all unresolved emotional issues will also be brought with us into the future. Just as the positive momentum of our positive actions and choices is kept moving forward through repetition (discipline), our negative karma based on our negative beliefs, thoughts and actions will be forwarded as limiting patterns in the future. Most people live in denial and self-delusion, or have blind spots when it comes to their destructive patterns. This is where the other laws of karma come into place and give us other opportunities to break through these patterns. It is good to know that the spirit is attracted to harmony and healing and will continue on the path of evolution.

THE SECOND LAW OF KARMA: THE LAW OF RECIPROCITY

If your feelings or actions toward someone are reciprocated, the other person feels or behaves in the same way toward you as you have felt or behaved toward him or her.

The Golden Rule
This is the foundation for the recommendation to love others as yourself. What you do unto others will be done to you. Treat others the way you would like to be treated, no matter how they are treating you.

The Platinum Rule
Treat others the way *they* want to be treated. This means you have to delve into their world and find out more about them.

The Boomerang Effect of Thoughts
Our thoughts and actions will come back to us like a boomerang. Sooner or later there will be a point when your actions and thoughts will return to you.

Suppose you are presented with a bill or invoice for damages because you've broken some goods from someone else. Here are the different ways you can pay your bill:

1. **Cash:** you feel the pain in your savings account right away. This is called *instant karma*.
2a. **Delayed short-term karma:** you pay with a credit card like American Express, Eurocard or Diner's Club and 30 days later (or sooner) you get the invoice.
2b. **Delayed long-term karma:** you charge it to your Visa or MasterCard and you can choose to pay only the minimum or in increments with interest, or all at once (2a).
3. **Delinquent long-term karma:** you opt for a delinquent account which will give you a bad credit history. This means that the 'punishment' you choose may be so far into the future that you may not even remember why you are being punished!

Personally I prefer the 'instant karma', because it is so easy to see the cause and effect. The more you evolve, the more you will have 'instant karma'.

The law of reciprocity also applies to positive karma. Sometimes you get an immediate return on your investment in a lump sum. Sometimes you get returns spread out over time; at other times you will not see returns until far into the future.

A word of warning: the law of reciprocity is not the only explanation for life's challenges. When we see someone who is suffering or is facing severe tragedy, we cannot assume that this is always the result of their own destructive choices in the past. Sometimes the soul takes on karma from others to relieve their suffering or as a service or an experience chosen to accelerate spiritual growth. The most important lesson is that we can never assume that if someone is suffering it is as a result of negative karma. Our intention should be to show love and compassion for everyone who is in their karmic process. If we don't, we also create new negative karma.

The law of reciprocity can give us an understanding of hardships, tragedies, suffering and premature death. The law of reciprocity is also the law of positive karma. All actions based on unconditional love, acts of kindness, services we perform or compassion we show others will come back to us. Just as old debts can accumulate interest, so can savings be multiplied.

Do we make choices for good, because that will bring us positive karma? Is that not selfish? All knowledge is karma: what use is knowledge if we choose not to act upon it? Ideally we should do good from the heart. When faced with some choices, it is OK to choose from an intellectual level for the benefits of doing the right thing. It is an added incentive in times of temptation. Gradually we will become more and more comfortable and more harmonious with making choices from the heart.

Conclusions

Some people use the law of reciprocity to become victims of their past selves and delve into feelings of guilt and shame. This law is meant to heal the past and change it. It gives us the possibility that our suffering is not in vain, that it serves the purpose of cleansing our memories and replenishing our systems with new energy. It makes us aware that we have to take responsibility for our lives.

There are many more laws that relate to karma. The two laws described here are the most important ones when it comes to understanding the relationship between karma and the emotions. For emotional balance, the added benefit of resolving past unresolved emotions is that each time we let go of a limiting memory, we are letting go of negative karma and creating more free emotional choice. *Free emotional choice is the way to positive karma.*

As we have read in this chapter, we can make choices from our mind or from our heart.

- **Hardware:** when we are at Level 1, we make our choices on a mental level, because that is good for us.
- **Heartware:** when we are at Level 2, we make our choices on a heart level, because they feel right (intuitive).
- **Software:** this is our spiritual core level (Level 3). We choose based on our spiritual guidance and follow the path of least resistance.

CHAPTER 5

EMOTIONAL BLOCKS TO HEALING

WE HAVE LOST OUR WAY AND BECOME FIXATED ON THE ILLUSION

Understanding sickness comes from understanding the wisdom of a healthy body. Disease is not something that happens to us; it is a part of an intricate system, telling us we need to make some changes in our approach to life. Every deviation from balance is imbalance. Imbalance is not the natural state for us, but that is where most people are. The reason is simple: lack of motivation coupled with lack of knowledge. Normally there is no knowledge needed to maintain health; everything we need is built into the system. By detaching ourselves from our divinity, however, we have detached ourselves from our self-regulating intelligence: the body's innate wisdom. So, now we have to re-learn what we already know, in order to take back what is already ours.

If we look at Nature, we see that when Nature is left alone there is an intelligence at work that keeps everything moving effortlessly. The circle of life happens naturally. We, as human beings, have chosen to disturb the rhythms of Nature and make life very complicated. We don't say what we mean to say, we worry about things we cannot change, we don't act on what we can change, we focus on what we don't have and we forget why we are here in the first place. Oops! We've got distracted by all the details that we created. We bought into the illusion of our own fantasy and have started believing it is real. It's like a child playing with toys: totally absorbed by them, he lives them, sees them and feels them. Our world is the same: full of toys that are there to make life more comfortable.

So what does all of this have to do with disease? The answer is: everything. You cannot isolate disease from the context in which it occurs. You cannot discount the world we live in; you cannot cure a disease without looking at the cause. If we understand the cause, we can really heal.

Emotional balance is about healing, which means solving the duality and become one perfect whole again. We are not yang *or* yin; both complement and balance each other perfectly.

WESTERN MEDICINE: LOOKING IN THE WRONG DIRECTION FOR A SOLUTION

Let's start with a short look at Western medicine, the epitome of science – or at least, that's what the orthodox medical establishment would have us believe.

Some missing links are:

- Doctors have lost the human touch (you are the next patient in line).
- No implementation of quantum physics and other breakthroughs in healing.
- Emphasis on symptoms and parts, not the whole.
- No real-time use of bio-energetics (the innate wisdom of the body).
- No place for the healing powers of the mind.
- Aversion to using nutri-ceuticals (nutritional therapy) and herbs; preference for chemical suppressing drugs.

Western medicine is unsurpassed when it comes to emergency medicine, especially in cases of trauma, acute circulatory or respiratory disorders and other life-threatening situations. When it comes to finding the true underlying cause of chronic disease, however, the whole picture is different.

ALTERNATIVE MEDICINE: LOST IN THE JUNGLE

This does not mean that alternative medicine is automatically the answer. I have studied alternative health therapies for over 30 years: acupuncture, homeopathy, herbalism, Qigong, hypnosis, flower essences, Reiki, therapeutic touch, osteopathic medicine, alternative cancer therapies, bio-energetic medicine, NLP, Shiatsu, orthomolecular therapy, Thalasso therapy, glandular therapy, chelation therapy, biofeedback and many more. My conclusion is that alternative medicine is a chaotic jungle. You need a guide to point you to the most appropriate therapy, and a practitioner best suited to your situation. It is not well organized. The principles, concepts and philosophies are impressive, and I will show you where all of this fits so you can understand the best steps to take. But the most important thing to remember is that you are in control of your own healing process, not the doctor or the therapist, whether he or she is 'alternative' or not.

HEALTH AND VITALITY

According to the World Health Organization, health is the state of being where an individual is free from emotional, physical and social suffering. In alternative medicine, a globally accepted definition of health is the optimal functioning of body, mind and soul. What I believe is that disease is not necessarily the opposite of health, but often a *consequence* of health. The body's innate intelligence, in its consistent and relentless pursuit of balance on all levels, will do what is necessary to maintain or create this balance. This is similar to keeping your house clean: you have to be consistent to maintain its upkeep. The question is: how many times a week do you tidy up? One person might do this constantly, another every other day, another once a week. Suppose you do it once a month; in that case there is so much to be done that you may be tired and exhausted afterwards, and for a few days to come.

Other important factors are: how many people live in the house? Whereabouts is the house (city, countryside, suburb)? How big is the house? How much pollution do the inhabitants generate? The body acts in a similar way: the amount of effort needed to maintain balance will depend on many factors. All of these can block healing:

- The amount of pollution coming in (alcohol, sugar, food additives, nicotine)
- The amount of residues going out (sweat, urine, stools, breath)
- How backlogged the system is (higher input than output of toxins)
- How much energy is diverted to other energy-consuming activities, such as stress, worries, infections, allergies, anxiety
- How much sleep you get (when we short-change ourselves on sleep, we have less capacity for detoxification and regeneration)
- How many 'building blocks' we have (antioxidants, vitamins, minerals, fatty acids, protein, carbohydrates)
- The amount and quality of fluids we take in
- The environment (if it's electromagnetically polluted or contaminated)
- The amount of infections (wars) going on in the body (for example: parasites, yeast infections, sinusitis, cavities, etc.)
- The amount of relaxation we get on a regular basis (meditation, music, etc.)
- The amount of exercise and movement we get
- The mental focus we have (how wired up we are for health or disease; this depends on our beliefs and thoughts)
- Our genetic constitution (inborn metabolic weaknesses and thoughts)
- The karmic baggage that we are dealing with right now.

So, being healthy is easy – just take control of all these factors and you are on your way! By the way, don't forget to reprogram your mind to condition it for vitality, longevity and optimal body functioning.

STOP LOSING LIFE-FORCE!

Of course, this is easier said than done; my purpose is, however, to help you with the most difficult aspect of this, and that is to take control of the biggest energy drain on your system. I think you know what I mean by now: *your emotional state*. This is the key ingredient in vitality, and yet is absent from most orthodox and alternative medical approaches.

Let's go to clinical practice and see this concept at work.

CASE STUDY

Jim was 68 years old. His face looked anguished and he had lost his usual smile. I had known Jim for over 15 years. I had seen him before when he came to me to treat his gout and weight problems. Jim was one of those patients who would only come when he had a serious problem. He would stick to any recommended change in lifestyle until it induced the desired changes, then go back to his old ways until he got into trouble again, then come back with a smile. He was the opposite of a hypochondriac: he would always pretend everything was perfect. His biggest vice was overeating; he loved 'all you can eat' restaurants and would let everybody know that these restaurants lost money on him. Of course he was overweight and had tried many diets unsuccessfully.

Looking at his facial expression that day, I knew something was awfully wrong. 'I have been diagnosed with cancer,' he said, 'they want to do surgery and radiation.' I was surprised and yet not surprised; I knew that sooner or later Jim would run into trouble. I had expected him to get heart problems. 'Where is the cancer?' I asked softly. 'Bladder cancer with metastasis to the bones,' he said and added: 'It's over. I know this is the end.' 'Why do you say that?' was my reply. 'I don't know, but I just know!' This was a new aspect of Jim I had not seen before. He was not a quitter, so I was really surprised. I thought there must be something else going on that I needed to find out about, some reason that had made him decide that there was no sense in fighting. *Shoganai* (acceptance of one's fate) is very useful when there really is nothing you can do, but it is not the same as defeat, which is detrimental when the situation is changeable. In cancer, *Shoganai* is part of the battle-plan, but not from the standpoint of defeat but from acceptance of the diagnosis. It means coming out of denial and accepting the challenge ahead. The diagnosis of cancer is the biggest hurdle, because of the hopelessness the diagnosis provokes in many people.

PLACEBO VERSUS NOCEBO

The following true story illustrates the power of the mind.

This happened over 36 years ago at the university hospital of Utrecht, where I studied medicine for six years. There are many examples of similar cases.

Two patients, both with the surname Jones and first initial W., were lying next to each other in the pulmonary ward. One had severe pneumonia and a painful cough; he was also an asthma sufferer. The other W. Jones was a chain smoker and had severe bronchitis; he was in hospital because he was coughing up blood and needed to get a bronchoscopy. The asthma patient Jones was diagnosed, after X-rays, with a very progressive and aggressive form of lung cancer; the prognosis was dim: six to nine months. The smoker Jones was told that his symptoms were of severe pneumonia, and he was put on a course of intravenous antibiotics and other appropriate medications. When he received the news, he was visibly relieved and his whole physiology changed. He was humming songs and telling jokes to the other patients. He was so happy because when he'd come into hospital he had been certain he had cancer and had given up hope; he had come to hospital with the belief that he was going to die. From that day he quit smoking and went back home to his life. The other W. Jones, as mentioned, was not so lucky; after having struggled for many years with chronic asthma, he was now diagnosed with metastatic lung cancer and was considered to be at the end of the road. He was terribly depressed and did not speak to anyone anymore. His family tried in vain to ease his despair, but could not change his funereal mood. Three months later this W. Jones passed away. The doctors were proven right once again in their predictions of the future.

However, the story does not end there: some weeks after asthma sufferer W. Jones' death, a medical student discovered that there had been a mix-up in the patient files. The surviving W. Jones, the former smoker, was the one who'd had the lung cancer all along. He was called back for another X-ray. To the great surprise of all the doctors there was no trace of lung cancer, except for a small calcification where the tumour had been. This W. Jones was completely cured and symptom-free.

This is a powerful example of what is known as the placebo effect, a strange medically unacceptable anomaly of the mind that states: 'If you believe strongly enough, you can be cured.' Of course it's not scientific; it's more esoteric or quasi-religious.

The deceased W. Jones, for his part, was a victim of *nocebo*, also a strange, medically unacceptable anomaly of the mind that states: 'If you believe strongly enough, you will become sick and even die.' When an authority such as a doctor has given you his or her prognosis, you absorb the information into your brain and your system. Most GPs forget that prognoses are based on statistics. Statistics are always on what's known as a Bell curve, which means there are always exceptions at both ends of the spectrum. So if the doctor tells you that you have six months to live, this can mean anywhere between two months and several years. If you die after six months precisely, you are a model patient and very suggestible. The doctor will be proved right. This is the 'nocebo' effect. If you refuse to be a statistic and can find the right mindset, other futures are possible.

So, let's go back to Jim. After talking to him, it became clear to me what was going on. Twenty-five years before, his wife had been diagnosed with cancer; she had known something was wrong with her breast for quite a while and was afraid she might have cancer. She delayed going to the doctor until she could no longer keep the problem hidden from Jim. She was diagnosed with breast cancer with metastasis to the bones. The doctors told her there was nothing they could do. Jim did not want to accept that. He sold some of his property and took her to a private clinic in Germany. She was operated upon and received radiation therapy and chemotherapy. Jim had taken leave of absence from his job and stood by her through the whole ordeal. He used up all his savings and got deeply in debt. She did not make it. She died after 10 months of struggle, exactly as the doctors had predicted. Jim never got over this and felt guilty: his guilt came from the idea that she had not trusted him enough to tell him what was going on. He was working hard at that time, had two jobs and his career was going very well. He had invested in real estate and, before her final fight, he had been very comfortable financially.

After the funeral Jim was a changed man: he started overeating and never shared his intimate feelings and thoughts with anyone.

Here was my diagnosis of Jim:

1. Unresolved emotions linked to guilt
2. A belief system that doctors were accurate in their prognosis about cancer
3. Underlying fear and depression preceding the development of cancer
4. Defeat and depression due to the diagnosis, coupled with a fear of death
5. Hostility toward God due to the unfairness of life.

EMOTIONAL ORGANS

In Traditional Chinese Medicine, every organ is known to resonate with a specific emotion.

Heart	Hurt, abandonment, disappointment, taking offence easily
Small intestine	Loneliness, oversensitivity, vulnerability
Bladder	Insecurity, indecisiveness, inability to let go
Kidneys	Fear, suspicion, distrust
Gallbladder	Frustration, irritation, bitterness
Liver	Anger, suppressed anger, jealousy, revenge
Lung	Depression, sadness, grief, loss, arrogance
Colon	Rigidity, dogmatic, defensiveness, perfectionism
Spleen/ Pancreas	Low self-esteem, despair, dependence on others
Stomach	Worry, anxiety, obsessiveness, disgust

In TCM there are also four 'organs' or energy systems which do not correspond to Western beliefs about the body, and they have exotic names: Triple Burner, Pericardium, Governor Vessel and Conception Vessel. They all correspond to the Fire element and are related to the neuroendocrine and immune systems.

The organs are divided according to the five elements, with corresponding vibrational rates. Some of these organ 'couples' are easily understood from a Western point of view, such as the liver and gallbladder, kidneys and bladder, pancreas and stomach. The less obvious combinations are: heart and small intestine, lungs and colon.

The elements and corresponding organ systems:

Fire	Heart, Small Intestine, Triple Burner, Pericardium
Earth	Spleen, Pancreas, Stomach
Metal	Lungs, Colon
Water	Bladder, Kidneys
Wood	Liver, Gallbladder
Neutral (void)	Governor Vessel, Conception Vessel

Each and every emotion will have a resonance with the energetic vibration of a specific organ or energetic system. This works in two ways: if the organ is weakened by any stressor, the person will become more prone to feel the corresponding emotion(s).

For example: a farmer exposed to toxic pesticides may develop problems with the liver. If the liver is out of balance, the farmer will gradually become more prone to irritation, frustration and anger. Little things may create big problems and the farmer will not understand why and become more and more impatient with co-workers, spouse and children. If there are many unresolved issues, these may come out. According to TCM, these unresolved issues will have predisposed the liver to be more vulnerable, and for that reason the pesticides will have had a greater effect than they otherwise would have had. In other words: unresolved issues make us more vulnerable and disease-prone. They also make us more accident-prone.

It's important to understand that if the organ is stressed or out of balance, if the underlying emotional causal factor is not resolved, balance will never be restored. The other side of the coin is: a person who is not dealing with a certain specific emotion will weaken the corresponding organ. We have discussed this in Chapter 2 when we spoke about hostility and the development of heart disease. When we are depressed, this will affect also the thymus gland and thus our immune system.

So, if you get angry with someone and you suppress this anger, you are inflicting damage to yourself. This may lead to a weakening of your liver function, which can result in the liver not being as efficient in eliminating toxins, which can result in you becoming chronically fatigued.

CASE STUDY

A dentist came to see me; I knew him from one of the seminars that I was teaching, which he'd attended. After the usual exchange of formalities and show of respect for each other's expertise, he explained to me that he had chronic hepatitis C. The normal Western treatment with interferon and steroids had failed, and he was afraid he'd end up with cirrhosis of the liver. *No better way to get what you don't want than feeding the fear of what you don't want.* After some soul-searching, it became apparent that he had some serious emotional problems with his father. His father had abused him as a child physically, and was a chronic alcoholic. After being diagnosed with cirrhosis of the liver, he'd undergone detox programmes and given up alcohol. Harry, the dentist, had not spoken with his father in over 12 years. He had told his wife that his father had died many years before. Three years previously, his father had called out of the blue and asked him for forgiveness. He had got very upset and yelled at his father that he would never forgive him. Shortly after that he was doing some dental surgery on a patient with hepatitis C and had got infected when he'd accidentally stuck a contaminated needle into himself. This had happened two days after his father's phone call. He knew immediately that he was infected and went the same day for medical help.

I asked Harry to look at this from another point of view: what he had yearned for all his life was to have a father. He and his father-in-law were close fishing buddies, but that is no substitute for being close to your own dad. I suggested to him that there could be a remote possibility that he had created this disease in order to face his biggest challenge: to let go of the past. I showed him, with a special alternative testing procedure, that if he did not forgive his father and let go of his anger, he would end up like his father, with cirrhosis of the liver.

Harry finally came to terms with the idea that the only true healing was letting go of the past and starting over. He did; not only was he completely cured of hepatitis C (very uncommon), he also developed a fantastic relationship with his father and they became the best of friends. What he discovered in that process was that they had much in common; much more than he could have ever imagined.

So, let's go back again to Jim: he had a disturbance of the water element (bladder cancer), and that relates to the following emotions: *insecurity, indecisiveness, not being able to let go and fear, mistrust, suspicion.* So Jim and I went to work (with the techniques I'll describe later in this book). Not only was Jim completely cured from bladder cancer and bone metastasis, but he healed so fast that his doctors were astonished. After three months there was only a tiny scar left in the bladder. The medical doctors, who had never before seen such a good response, told him that he was an exceptional patient and did not believe that the alternative treatment with herbs, vitamins and homeopathy had had anything to do with it. And they were absolutely right! I believe that the reason Jim got well (and has not had any recurrence after five years) is that he let go of the unresolved emotions of the past. His longing for 'all you can eat' places has also waned considerably. He still has the gout, but as long as that is not bothering him, I'm not likely to see him and that is, of course, his choice. The point is that emotional blocks are as ubiquitous as the air we breathe; everybody has them. Disease, discomfort and physical and mental suffering are just ways to get our attention on dealing with this burden of karma we carry with us.

Freeing Your Demons

Every illness is an opportunity to overcome some demon from the past and let go of something that no longer serves us. When we free ourselves from our self-induced demons, we rebound and have more vitality and more to live for. Any attempt to cure anything without looking at the real cause is another way to lock the past even deeper into our subconscious programs. By 'solving' our problems with chemical drugs, we are asking for more serious problems in the future. In other words: every attempt at a cure that does not respect the body's own intelligence is a potential risk. True healing only happens when the unconscious causal factors are found and dealt with. *Everything else is just treating the symptoms.*

OMEGA HEALING

Let's look some more at the origins of disease.

Body, mind and spirit cannot be separated from each other. Our thoughts play an important role in directing the flow of energy. After studying more than 80 different forms of alternative healing in depth, I decided to combine the most effective aspects of these different modalities into one system: *Omega Healing*.

The basic premise of Omega Healing is that most diseases are created on a subconscious level. This has nothing to do with what many people do – namely, blaming themselves for becoming ill. That is neither relevant nor the case. We do not consciously choose to create disease, nor do we enjoy the process of suffering. We cannot do this on command – at least, most of us can't – nor can we change it just by deciding we want out. It is far more complicated than that. If you bear with me, you will get some important insights into this. Disease or symptoms are the means to an end. It was never our *intent* to create suffering. What we really wanted was maybe some attention, respect, admiration, care, trust and other aspects of being loved. Maybe we were tired of all the heavy responsibilities we'd taken on our shoulders and we got ourselves into a 'killer loop' of negative thoughts. Maybe we were not happy with our jobs, relationships or our lives, and just wanted out. Maybe we wanted to protect ourselves from unwanted attention. Maybe we overreacted and were too overzealous, and wanted out without losing face. Maybe we did not know another way to keep from destroying ourselves, or maybe we believe we don't deserve to be successful or loved or wealthy or healthy. Maybe we feel we needed punishment.

DISEASE FROM LEVEL 1 OF CONSCIOUSNESS

Most people create disease from the first level of consciousness; it takes years of hard work and neglecting yourself. Years of negative beliefs and self-defeating self-talk. We work hard at getting sick while running around not feeling anything else. Take a good look around you and you will see the masses moving in this direction. It is like a river flowing in the direction of the waterfall. There is nothing you can do to turn it around; it is unstoppable. That is where most people are: part of that river of ignorance heading toward their downfall.

DISEASE FROM LEVEL 2 OF CONSCIOUSNESS

Another large group of people create disease from the second level of consciousness; it takes months or even years of not feeling well and ignoring your inner voice and intuition. You knew you should not have taken this new job; it pays more but the cut-throat environment makes you dread going to the office every day. Many of us keep motivating ourselves with money, career advancement, prestige, goodies (perks). We know that a relationship has no future; we hope for years that our partner will change, losing precious life energy in the process.

There are many examples of incongruous behaviour, where we have strong feelings but we elect to ignore them. We sometimes become 'hooked' on people or objects in a way that causes us to lose our own identity and disconnect from our feelings and intuition, and as a consequence we sap our life-force. It is not easy being honest to yourself (I speak from experience) and let go of harmful attachments and toxic people. *Disharmony searches for disharmony.* In the end it does not matter if you believe that we create our reality or not. Consciously most of us cannot control what happens to us, but we can choose the way we deal with it. Also, it should be clear and obvious that unless the negative emotions, beliefs, thoughts, feelings and/or negative use of one's personal power are released, the energy leaks will continue. Then, sooner or later, illness may result.

Healing is about restoring balance on all levels. That also means exercise (movement), eating a nutritious balanced diet, meditation (relaxing), stress management, lifestyle changes, losing or gaining weight (whatever is needed), changes in mental attitude and so on.

EMOTIONS AND THEIR EFFECTS ON THE BODY

Every thought or emotion has bio-energetic resonance: this travels through the body at the speed of light and is picked up by the chakras and meridians. Biochemical signals (neurotransmitters) affect all the cells and tissues. Thoughts and other oscillations are sent to the space around us and beyond. These can be picked up by others. We vibrate with information; we are thinking and feeling bio-energetically active bodies. By addressing only one aspect of this system, we fail to influence all parts of the body.

One of the most important keys to healing is how people deal with the body's signals. What is their attitude toward health and their bodies? Do they feel they are in control, or are there feelings of despair and helplessness? Everything that happens to us has meaning; we can change this meaning with new information.

Jim believed that doctors were always right. He had one very painful reference point for this belief, and filtered out all information contradicting it. It was my job to change that belief and offer him a new meaning. The next step was for him to release his guilt, fear and anger. By creating harmony inside, he was able to withstand radiotherapy easily and recover more quickly than other patients.

To summarize this in another way: the patient has to be *congruent with healing*. The patient should be dealing with all the emotional issues that underlie his or her problem. Patients should accept that they stand a reasonable chance of victory. If they can follow their body's innate healing intelligence, healing will occur much more often and much more effortlessly.

HEALING MODALITIES

Let's look at the four broad categories of healing.

1. Mechanical Medicine (Level 1 Consciousness)

Doctors try to suppress disease with chemicals, surgery, radiation, organ transplants, artificial organs and other means. This is the level of hard work; it requires knowledge, specialized training and years of study. Many mistakes are made because the therapies can be very toxic to even healthy subjects. This should be the last resort. Herbal medicine is a softer choice here and is not as toxic, but also requires dedicated study by the practitioner.

2. Bio-energetic Medicine (Level 1 to Level 2 Consciousness)

Most of the alternative therapies, such as acupuncture, homeopathy, flower essences and Reiki, fall into this category. By working on the energetic systems, they try to assist the body in healing. Many ways have been discovered to communicate with the body's own intelligence, such as biofeedback, applied kinesiology, face diagnosis, tongue diagnosis, pulse diagnosis, electro-diagnosis. Some therapists work more on an intuitive level; others work more from a systematic approach. Depending on their approach, they are acting at Level 1 or Level 2 of consciousness.

3. Psychosomatic Medicine (Level 1 and Level 2 Consciousness)

The starting point here is that body and mind are one. More and more therapies are being used to influence the mind. In this category we have therapies such as hypnosis, self-hypnosis, yoga, meditation, subliminal audiotapes, affirmations and visualizations.

4. Intention Medicine (Level 3 Consciousness)

This is healing from a distance. One of the best examples is prayer. Another is hands-on healing. Prayer has been proven to have an effect. One of the leading authorities on this subject is Dr Larry Dossey, MD. He has written several bestsellers; one of his best is *Be Careful What You Pray For, You Might Just Get It*. In this book he looks at the flipside of healing prayer, exploring the unintentional harm we can cause with our thoughts, prayers and wishes. The conclusion is clear: we must assume a greater level of responsibility for our negative and hurtful thoughts. There is a great deal of evidence of the power of intention, especially when multiplied by the collective mind of many believers. Prayer is communicating with the collective consciousness; it can work for or against us. If prayer is a confirmation of your pain, poverty or misery, it will only reinforce what you don't have. When we pray from the heart with love, it will be from a different level.

The most important lesson to be learned is to *be very clear and specific in your intent*. Your intent is the spearhead of your energy which will be multiplied by the collective resonance of all your past and future intentions. To put it in simpler words: most people who are sick are more preoccupied with what they *don't* want than with what they *do* want. Their focus on their fears creates images that are the opposite of what they really want. These images are then the intent they send out in time and space.

In neuroscience they say that the subconscious mind cannot hear the word '*no*'. I believe this is not entirely correct. The subconscious mind is predominantly visual and will create an image of what you are focusing on. So you will actually see an image of what you don't want; for that reason your subconscious believes that you want what you are projecting on your internal 'screen'!

I remember the following incident that happened to me about 12 years ago when I was living in California; this was before I understood about the three levels of consciousness. One day I had the feeling that I would get into a car accident. I could not get rid of this feeling. I started to drive very carefully. (When I was 21 years old I had been in intensive care with an injury that resulted from a serious car accident.) Nevertheless, some three months later I did get into a minor accident when my car slipped from the road and hit a tree. There was only some slight damage to the bumper of the car. I felt relieved and happy with that accident. Never before was I so happy about damage to my car. Years later I had a recurrence of that same feeling, but the difference was that now I was prepared. Instead of focusing on what I did *not* want, I started to focus on what I wanted: to get home safely with my car intact. Gradually the feeling disappeared, and I have not been in a car accident since.

The more you evolve to Level 3, the faster these manifestations occur. This can be very scary. Sometimes you get an idea and, before you know it, someone pops up in your life who can help you carry out and manifest that idea. That is the power of intention; it is like nuclear power and something we need to use wisely. It is like having a magic wand that instantly manifests your thoughts, desires and wishes. Then you'd better watch out what you think. Each thought had better be a loving thought, because it will have an impact. This is already happening whether you are on Level 3 or not. There may be a bigger time delay between intention and manifestation, and the effects may or may not be as strong but, over time, all our intentions leave an eternal imprint.

YOUR HEALING JOURNEY

I am sure that you get the picture. Every healing journey should start with a clear intent on getting well and relieving the body of all negative intents of the past. If it is attention you want, your intent should be to get attention in a healthy way. If you subconsciously yearn for respect, you should know that by giving it unconditionally to others, the law of karma will sooner or later bring it back to you. Needless to say, it is more worth your while to satisfy all your needs while being healthy. The question we need to answer is: what was the original positive intent behind my illness? In what other way, using my current knowledge of karma, can I pull what I need into my reality while remaining healthy and vital?

CHAPTER 6

CHAKRAS: GATEWAYS TO THE SOUL

In this chapter I will discuss one of the most important ways we can shift our focus from our physical desires, needs and pains to our quantum body – and, thereby, increase our level of consciousness. Our quantum body is the larger-than-life energetic hologram that is the expression of our spirit and consciousness. Your quantum body will determine who and what you attract into your life.

Let's look first at the way the chakras and meridians function in connection with how we send and receive information, and what the ramifications are for our spiritual path. In his book *Science and Human Transformation*, William A. Tiller, PhD, describes research done on humans with specific instruments that can detect electromagnetic (EM) radiation. What he discovered is that EM energy radiates from the body as a result of a variety of complex processes such as atomic shifts, physical rotations, vibrations of the molecules, movement of the cell membranes, pulsation of organs and body movement in general. The larger the entity causing this displacement, the lower the EM frequency. His conclusion is that the body can be seen as a type of transmitter with a receiving antenna. Incoming EM waves of a particular frequency will activate the body's organs or tissues that resonate with that frequency. What is interesting is that if there is no harmonious correlation between the movements of the body parts, there is no integration and the out-flowing radiation has no discernible pattern.

In other words: disharmony emits disharmonious information. The opposite is also true: the greater the degree of correlated movements between the different organs and tissues, the more harmonious the patterns will be and the greater their information content. So it's in our best interests to synchronize all of our bodily systems to create greater integration and harmony.

Incongruence, confusing thoughts, blame and guilt all contribute to chaos and disharmony in our system. Dr Tiller has found different key EM output levels, which he correlates with the following distinct sources: physical, ethereal, astral (emotional), the instinctive mind, the intellectual mind, the spiritual mind and the spirit. Each of these domains is unique and sends out information at a different frequency. There is a progressive increase in velocity, and this corresponds with higher and more subtle domains.

These output levels correspond with the chakras. As we go higher up in the body, we get into more subtle energies. According to Dr Tiller, the autonomic nervous system (ANS) has the capacity to be a receiving antenna. The ANS influences the endocrine glands, heart, respiration, circulation, peristalsis and more. It also serves as an excellent wave-guide through the nerves to a multitude of end-points just under the surface of the skin. These acupuncture points (APs) are thus sometimes considered a set of 'antenna elements' in this system. These sensitive points number in the thousands, and owing to that number their capabilities exceed the most advanced radar system available today. Yes, you read that correctly: you are one of the most sensitive pieces of equipment on Earth, much more advanced than anything humanity could ever make. You could detect a stealth bomber on the other side of the world with your eyes closed. The other fact you should know is that the human body's antenna system can function over a wide range of wavelengths and produces a scanner beam with a wide range of detection.

The APs are measurable with sensitive equipment. One of the key conclusions reached by Dr Tiller was that the primary structural elements of the acupuncture system are located at the ethereal level rather than at the physical level. This explains why there is no major histological difference between APs and the surrounding tissue. In other words, APs differentiate themselves by their different energetic vibrations from surrounding skin. Or to state it more simply: APs are connected to an energetic system other than normal skin. They are, instead, part of an intricate complex bio-energetic regulatory system linked to the chakras. What is clear is that the acupuncture meridians allow us to connect and create communications between the internal physical and subtle substances of the body with our environment and other beings from our species. At the ethereal level this network can be said to represent the 'subtle nadi' of the ancient Hindu teachings. It is probable that even more subtle levels of energy and substance are involved in this antenna system. This brings us back to the chakra system, which is intertwined with the endocrine glands. The endocrine glands, via the hormones, control all the chemical factories of the body. The chakras-endocrine system transduces energy from the subtle level to the physical level. The chakras are linked to our past (our biography) and also to our current attitudes (thinking); this is translated into our biology.

Chakras also connect us with our soul template. The purpose of the soul is to attract situations and people who have created similar unresolved conflicts from the past, so we get the chance to resolve them from a more evolved moment in our evolutionary process.

Based on Dr Tiller's excellent research, we can now expand further on the chakras and their meaning. The chakras are an integral part of the Eastern spiritual tradition. Medical intuitive Carolyne Myss, a bestselling author, explains in her book *Anatomy of the Spirit* the correlation between the chakras and the ten *serifot* of the Jewish Kabbalah and the seven sacraments of the Catholic church. These ten qualities have traditionally been organized into seven levels. The qualities attributed to each of the seven levels are virtually identical with those of the chakras. Myss says: 'Learning to embody these qualities while facing life's challenges is the essence of the spiritual journey.'

Viewing illness and crises as a chance to exercise these spiritual truths brings a level of meaning to the experience that accelerates healing. In the chakras, any new information is compared to our old, unresolved issues and the body is directed in a certain direction that will allow us to confront those issues or otherwise resolve them.

Our subconscious mind is programmed to look for stability,

security, love and the status quo. Change is not welcome; it is a threat to the status quo. To be able to welcome change and challenges is a learned behaviour; it is not automatic. That is why so many children have a problem with their parents leaving home and go through the whole ordeal from crying to throwing tantrums to the dismay of millions of babysitters and nannies. The subconscious also helps us to create what we think of a lot and will attract in your life the things on which you focus. If you desire a lot of money because you are afraid of poverty, you are focused on avoiding poverty and may never become wealthy or stay stuck in the poverty consciousness of needing more and more. As long as there is a discrepancy between what we want consciously and what we fear subconsciously, we will have a duality that will drain our energy and create sabotage. This can eventually result in illness and suffering. The chakras respond less to emotions but more to the processes or patterns we are in; they correspond to the different sublevels of consciousness. We will review them one by one; by familiarizing ourselves with them, we will recognize many things of ourselves and this may help you to create the transformations needed to change your life permanently.

ANATOMY OF THE CHAKRAS

Through the chakras, our higher self can manifest a part of itself in time and space. The spirit is boundless, unlimited and not confined to time and space; it needs a gateway in matter to manifest itself. These gateways work both ways; we can use them to access the spirit. Each of the main chakras represents a state of consciousness; they are complementary and influence each other. When we block our life-force, we also block our chakras, and then old patterns come to the surface; we get stuck, become compulsive, fanatic, helpless, etc. The chakras control our behaviour and thinking. Getting insights into the cause of our problems or harmonizing the energy focus in our body allows us to let go of the past and the consequential cyclical thoughts, and our life-force reasserts itself.

Each chakra has a tremendous creative and manifesting power; the question is: do we have full access to the use of their potential?

The degree of our accessibility depends on several factors such as the spiritual degree of insight we have achieved in previous existences, our programming in this life (education, parents or environment), our current environment (the people we surround ourselves with) and our commitment to spiritual growth. The most important key ingredient determining our ability to manifest is not the past; all those past issues can be overridden by consciously focusing on empowering ways to deal with the turbulence we face day to day. In other words: by focusing on the now and deciding consistently to go to your heart and let go, you can harness the powers of your chakras. Important in this concept is that the past continues to repeat itself through our lives to give us the opportunity to heal and let go. By doing that we stop from being in repetitious cycles and make progress rapidly to higher states of awareness and consciousness.

The chakras filter the amount of energy from our unlimited source to reduce it to what we can use right now and to keep us focused on the current issues. Opening up the chakras allows access to much more information and a move up the ladder toward being multi-sensorial. To free ourselves and to reach the euphoric state of unconditional happiness which is the prerequisite for unconditional love and total surrender, we need to become aware of our own imaginary boundaries. These boundaries are protective fences around us, based on our fears. We will need to get access to our courage to break through and expand our reality. To harmonize our chakras is to heal ourselves of old constricting or self-destructive patterns.

We will now define the chakras one by one and get more ideas on how to use them to our advantage.

CHAKRA 1 (*MULADHARA*): ROOT OR BASE CHAKRA

This chakra is located at the base of the spine (your coccyx).

This chakra has the lowest vibrational rate and is connected with matter. Matter is symbolic of the Source that feeds us and takes care of us. It's about survival. All time-space events are connected to our existence on planet Earth. This chakra holds the blueprint for our physical manifestation: bones, muscles, skin, hair, nails and blood vessels. It relates to bodily support: the base of the spine, legs, feet and the immune system. It becomes disrupted when we are not feeling safe or when we live in continuous fight-or-flight mode. We then get stuck in a mode that will be fixated long after the danger has passed. That explains why many people who have experienced poverty first-hand seek security by collecting more and more material goods.

Taking care of ourselves starts with knowing where we stand and consciously making choices about where we want to be, and then taking the necessary action. If we either neglect our base for survival or get obsessed by it, we will never tap into our full potential of consciousness. The result is to overemphasize good looks, status, prestige, possessions and career – but if we do this we will never experience the fruits of unconditional happiness.

Chakra 1 constantly provides us with information about our body's functioning. By tuning in to our body's language we can serve its needs and create harmony that will improve our quality of life and longevity. We will learn to handle stress properly and ground ourselves to create a sense of stillness or calm.

The organs most associated with the first chakra are the adrenals and the colon. The adrenals act as our 'fight or flight' system which responds automatically in situations of stress, shock or panic. The essence here is to become true to one's path and not be ruled by what others say. Self-respect, a sense of personal honour and letting go of guilt and fears from the past feed strong positive energy to the root chakra. The first chakra asks us to honour the family/ tribe into which we were born, even if life's journey has pushed us to move on. To take this one step further, we all have the same mother, which is our planet. There is a correlation between how we treat ourselves and how we treat Mother Earth. When we pollute, exhaust, overuse, abuse, poison, disrespect and are negligent with our physical bodies, this creates dissonance in the root chakra. This is exactly how we treat Mother Earth. We can also see, looking at our economy, that it is based on survival mode, the relentless pursuit of accumulating more and more. Competitive happiness is the main survival mechanism. For us to survive as a species and to thrive, we have to learn how to live in harmony with our planet. The first step is for us to harmonize our root chakra. Each step that we take toward a higher consciousness will have an effect on the collective consciousness of humanity.

Raising Chakra 1 Awareness

Two of the main patterns that chakras create are based on a fear of change. Change is a threat to survival. This can lead to a fear of success and a fear of rejection.

Success is not a goal but is a result of a growth process. Success is the degree of fulfilment that results when we commit to our values. If we don't, the perceived success will be hollow and not satisfying; it will become part of our competitive happiness, which, as we've learned, is not happiness at all. Valuing ourselves means committing to our need for growth, and this will bring success to every aspect of our lives. We need to learn to forgive ourselves and love ourselves, and accept our mistakes as part of growing up and also as part of a collective system where we help each other's growth by being ourselves. To raise the manifestation and creative powers of chakra 1, we need to become process-oriented instead of results-oriented. The goal is not even the most important determining factor of our success; instead it is the person we become in pursuit of that goal. When we 'fail', we need to look inside to search for the positive intent of our lack of success. Is it a way to get attention, care or another basic need met? Do we prefer to stay in our comfort zone? Do we really want the goal we have chosen? Do we do it for ourselves or to prove ourselves to others?

Here are some key ingredients to consider:

- Success comes from dealing with the unwanted side-effects in a harmonious manner.
- Success is embracing your talents and skills but also your limitations and weaknesses (your identity).

- Success means confronting your deepest fears and overcoming them by accepting them.
- Success is becoming congruent with your values and basing your goals on that.
- Success means accepting that others will criticize you, hold you back and/or limit your personal growth, and choosing instead what *you* want (change is also a threat to your environment).
- When success is one-sided and we are not successful in other areas (relationships, parenthood, health), we sabotage ourselves and we need to refocus on the areas that need our attention and learn to deal with the associated fears and issues.
- It is only when we learn to deal with and accept rejection and failure that we can become really successful.
- Success based on a win–lose concept is negative karma and the ultimate failure.
- Success on the highest level of consciousness is achieved when the journey is effortless and when in that process many others are elevated to a higher state of consciousness.

Chakra 1 Disharmony

When chakra 1 is out of balance we will see more of: superficial opinions, formalities, pride, self-criticism, perfectionism, stinginess, pettiness and narrow-mindedness. Also we'll see attachment to dogma, rules, structure and organization, and an express preference for secrets, mysteries, ceremonies, rituals, suspicions and superstitions.

- ***Qualities to be developed:*** letting go, connecting with the universal consciousness, tolerance, softness, team spirit, humbleness and love
- ***Archetypes connected with chakra 1:*** the organizer, entrepreneur, engineer, architect, accountant, bookkeeper.

Chakra 1 Overview

Elements	Matter, Earth
Organs	Rectum, colon, adrenals, stress, bones, legs, blood vessels, immune system
Consciousness	Survival, security, bodily functions, adaptation to change
Harmony	Trust, self-respect, letting go, acceptance, feeling safe
Disharmony	Humiliation, shame, abuse of authority, feeling inferior
Sacred truth	All is one
Sacrament	Baptism: welcoming into life, family and community
Energy content	Tribal power
Fears	Fear of change, fear of rejection
Special	Feed the body with nutritious foods and thoughts
Emphasis	Competitive happiness: success
Affirmations	'It is safe for me...' 'I am able...' 'I have...'

CASE STUDY: CHAKRA 1

She entered my office and it was as if she were dressed for a fashion show. Lucy was a classical homeopath – that is, an alternative health professional working with a very specific therapy based on the patient's personality and his or her specific expression of symptoms. She was very well-known and highly respected in the homeopathy field and had written two books on the subject. She was around 40 years old and good-looking. Everything on her looked as if it were made specifically to emphasize her beauty. She had a lot of gold jewellery, from six bracelets to eight gold rings, some with diamonds. She drove an expensive sports car and everything around her was aimed at creating the impression of success and an eye for detail. I had seen her on several of my workshops; she was always on her own and did not mingle much with the others. I had spoken with her and she was very shy, never looking me directly in the eye. I was really puzzled about why she had come to see me; on the phone she'd sounded urgent and told me she was desperate. After the initial opening formalities, I asked her how I could help her. 'I have terrible hair loss and I am really worried I will lose all my hair.' When I took a closer look I could indeed see that, despite the first impression that her hair was OK, she had a serious alopecia (hair loss) problem. When I questioned her about her medical history, a whole array of medical problems came out: when she was 16 years old she had become obsessed with her weight and suffered from bulimia and anorexia nervosa. She took laxatives because of her constipation, but the underlying cause was that her diet was terrible. She ate biscuits or crackers with no butter, sometimes with a tiny bit of fruit or a tomato. At dinner she would eat a piece of chicken with some vegetables. She was hypo-metabolic (slow functioning of the thyroid), which is normal for someone with her eating habits. She had also had surgery for melanoma (skin cancer) over 10 different times. She had her own sunbed at home and, despite doctor's orders, she would still tan three times a week to 'look good'. She was fair-skinned and blonde and had a predisposition for melanoma. She also suffered on and off with sciatica on the left side, especially during menstruation. To top it all off, she was a workaholic: she worked 14 to 15 hours a day seeing patients, six days a week.

When we did tests of her adrenals, they were completely overworked. That was the cause of her fatigue and insomnia. I started with my diagnostic work-up, which included blood tests to check adrenal function, vitamin and mineral levels and normal blood work. I also used *applied kinesiology*, which is also known as muscle-testing. Muscle-testing is a simple and non-invasive process that allows doctor and patient to work together in a way that communicates with the innate intelligence of the body. A specific muscle is tested while I ask the patient a question. This is always a yes/no question. If a muscle that originally tests strong or firm changes in strength, this usually indicates a 'yes'. If the muscle strength stays the same, that means 'no'. The beauty of this system is that it can give you insights into the body's functioning in just a few minutes. In serious cases we always have to back this up with other forms of diagnosis.

What made Lucy's case even more interesting was that the only significant thing I found was the blockage of the first chakra. At first I did not believe it, and tested her in other ways, but the results came out the same. At that time I was not as familiar with the symptoms of the chakras. I grabbed a manual for a seminar I attended run by Dr Susan Brennan, a chiropractor in California, on Emotional Body Integration. Dr Brennan teaches seminars on balancing the chakras. Here I saw the list of physical complaints related to imbalance of the first chakra: haemorrhoids, constipation, weight problems, sciatica, anorexia nervosa, skin and hair problems, adrenal insufficiency. It was as if I were reading Lucy's medical history. I sat down with her and started to probe into her past.

Now, one of the most powerful ways to damage the first chakra is being abused and humiliated. What came out was that she had married her first boyfriend, whom we shall call Pete. She had been with Pete since she was 17 years old, and married him when she was 20 years old. Pete had always dominated the relationship and she had been humiliated by him in public and at home. He was constantly criticizing her and nothing she did was right. She could not cook, he said, her bottom was too big and her breasts too small. She had silicone implants to please him and now he was demanding she get bigger implants. After the first time she'd had implants, he'd resumed having sex with her for a few months after a hiatus of six years. She also knew he'd had an extramarital affair and felt humiliated by that. He also physically and verbally abused her. I asked her why she did not leave him. 'I am afraid. He is the only man I have ever trusted. I know what I have now.' It sounded almost unbelievable: this beautiful young woman, with a successful career and everything else going for her, was afraid to leave this man who was so bad for her self-esteem. When I tested her on her identity, she tested weak with being herself, which is an indication of not accepting oneself. She tested strong when she said: 'I am Pete,' an indication of wanting to please him at all costs. In another book by Carolyn Myss, I found that she relates ME (Chronic Fatigue Syndrome) to an energetic disturbance of the first chakra in people who feel very vulnerable and insecure. These people try to be all things to all people and they finance too many people and/or projects with their energy; as a result, their immune system collapses, which can lead to cancer. Another important point is that because Lucy had become totally dependent upon her husband, all her energy circuits had become attached to him. This imbalance generally results in a woman having no energy to keep her own body healthy, and simultaneously generates in her husband a feeling of being 'smothered'.

Based on this information, I asked her if her husband had hair-loss problems. She said 'yes' and added that he had a problem accepting he was going bald. Now the picture was complete: Lucy had a severely dysfunctional first chakra with, as a result, her focus on looks, earning money and security. Divorcing Pete was too big a change and presented her with too many unknowns. All her physical complaints were related to the first chakra as well.

Lucy's therapy was not easy: she expected some sort of ongoing acupuncture, vitamin and homeopathy treatment. I told her that first she needed to do some visualization and affirmation work to balance the first chakra. These are the two affirmations she had to do while stimulating the special acupuncture points I will teach you about in Part II (the kidney and bladder points, which deal with fear and insecurity):

- **General affirmation for balancing chakra 1** (using kidney acupoints): 'I feel completely safe and relaxed and I can let go of past hurts easily, now and continuously.'
- **Personal affirmation for Lucy** (using bladder acupoints): 'I am able to accept myself and love myself just the way I am and I feel good and secure, even when Pete criticizes or rejects me, now and continuously.'

That doesn't sound like very complicated, does it? She was to repeat each affirmation six times a day while massaging the corresponding points and visualizing her body full of light and her hair fully restored.

Lucy rang me up two weeks later, completely excited: 'Roy, I decided to get a divorce and I am moving out next week – I already have a house!' I was impressed with how quickly this had worked, and decided to start looking seriously into these things called chakras. Lucy in the meantime is doing great, and has no hair-loss and no recurrence of the skin cancer; she is taking dance classes and is going out with someone who is very nice to her.

CHAKRA 2 (*SVADISTHANA*): SACRAL CHAKRA

This is located in the lower abdomen, around the bladder area. The consciousness is focused on expression and creativity. This chakra is of a higher vibrational rate than chakra 1, and this is where enjoyment and pleasure comes in. Using the comparison of a baby, the first need is to be fed; once the hunger is satisfied and survival ensured, the baby will start to enjoy itself, making sounds, looking around, finding objects to touch, taste and so on. Matter in movement becomes soft and pliable. The associated element is water. Water is the crystal that holds the memory of the original hologram. Water is also symbolic of fluidity, expression, flexibility, adaptation. This chakra controls the body's liquids: lymph, blood, phlegm, sperm, urine, sweat, saliva, the viscous liquid of the eyes, mucous membranes.

The parts of the body most affected by the second chakra are: the reproductive organs, large intestine, pelvis and lower pelvic area, including the hip area. This chakra's energy becomes disrupted by stifled creative energy, money and sexual conflicts, power struggles, lack of joy in one's daily routines, such as dead-end relationships or jobs, and control tactics that are not based on the first karmic law of 'Honour One Another'. To accept and acknowledge all of our feelings and to realize that acceptance does not mean being stuck with them or responding based on these feelings. We get stuck in memories of the past and keep responding in non-empowering patterns. That explains why many people will suppress their feelings and feel guilty for enjoying themselves. At this level it is important to learn how to deal constructively with our feelings and emotions. Consciousness can only exist when we are in touch with our feelings; these feelings keep us in the 'here and now awareness' and help us distinguish between what attracts and what distracts. The mind needs feelings in order to direct energy to the areas where it is needed. In diseases where there is numbness or paralysis such as Hansen's disease (leprosy), the physical body gets mutilated and scarred. The more we develop our consciousness, the more we can feel and the more nuances and distinctions we can make – and the clearer any incoming messages will be.

Through this chakra we can lay the foundation for transcending to the multi-sensorial and developing our intuition. We learn to distinguish what our feelings are, where they come from and what the causal patterns and unresolved issues are. The second chakra is our joy centre; when developed we can develop our instinct for finding the path that will give us the most joy. When we are stuck we will meet with one emotional roadblock after another, or we may seek joy in substances and situations such as drugs or junk food.

On this same level, but based on trauma, people can be stuck in a mode of prostituting their life-force. This can manifest in actual prostitution, abusive relationships, incest, rape and physical abuse. Always keep in mind that we are receivers and senders of energetic information that will be picked up by others tuned in to the same wavelength. Many people become aware sooner or later that they are stuck in a disempowering situation and that they are losing their precious life-force and emotional balance. They are locked into relationships that are abusive, destructive and disempowering to them. Controlling others and letting yourself be dominated are two sides of the same coin. One cannot exist without the other; they are yin and yang.

Some of the ailments associated with chakra 2 disharmony and fear of losing control or authority are: breast cancer, lower back pain, prostate or ovarian cancer, uterus ailments and cancer, impotency, frigidity and bladder problems.

To find balance in ourselves so we can learn to respect and honour others' boundaries and accept them as they are instead of trying to change, manipulate or control them, even with good intentions, will harmonize the second chakra. When it comes to sexuality, it is important to be aware that we do not dissociate from our innermost feelings. By opening up and connecting on all levels, we open up to more joy and freedom of expression. When we experience inhibition of sexual enjoyment this is seldom organic but usually comes from fear of expressing emotion. When we connect to our hearts and open up all the blocked channels, this will deepen our levels of enjoyment. Being able to enjoy and experience passion, ecstasy and happiness is essential to our spiritual growth.

Respect Your Feelings

Respecting ourselves means acknowledging and accepting our feelings and emotions. Only when we accept the bad feelings as well as the good, without judging or fear of being overwhelmed, can we avoid blockages. We can learn to *feel good about feeling bad* through owning the process we are in without suppressing anything. Feelings help us to connect to the different chakras and maintain a circulation of energy. Being able to deal harmoniously with the whole range of our feelings is the foundation of emotional balance. Emotions are the connection between our inner world and the outer world. In order to share joy, harmony and love with others, we need to find these things and cultivate them in ourselves and until they become second nature.

Raising Chakra 2 Awareness

Due to the higher vibrational rate of the second chakra, it becomes the place where we can start detaching ourselves from the illusionary realm called matter and objective reality. Another area that chakra 2 can help with is detaching from other patterns: for example, being a victim, being in a dissatisfying job, relationship, addictive cycle and so on. The key is to move on when there is nothing more to learn from a current pattern. The greatest growth is achieved by breaking free of that pattern. Someone who is stuck in chakra 2 can use techniques such as meditation, mantras, chanting and affirmations to detach from their feelings.

CASE STUDY

During a week-long retreat on meditation conducted by Deepak Chopra in Goa (India), I met a 38-year-old woman who had undergone surgery a few times for uterine problems. I was surprised to hear that she meditated eight hours a day. When she was experiencing marital problems, she told me she'd meditate even more. 'Why?' I asked. She said, 'It helps me detach and Chopra says that meditation helps to burn your karma.' She had been practising meditation for over eight years. I explained to her she had taken what Dr Chopra said out of context to serve her own purpose: avoiding her true feelings. I also explained to her that she was afraid of losing control and, by not having sex with her husband, she was creating new karma by keeping him and herself in a dysfunctional relationship. I told her that by fleeing into meditation she was not burning karma, but creating negative karma. Through our sessions together she gained more insight into how to deal with her situation. I gave her two choices:

1. Commit to the relationship and burn negative karma by confronting all unresolved issues and emotions that would come up.
2. Stop the relationship and burn negative karma by confronting all the ramifications of abandonment, fear of being alone, fear of not finding another man.

This story illustrates the danger of misusing meditation to avoid reality: eventually your issues will catch up with you and manifest themselves as physical problems or other painful experiences. The true meaning of detachment is not the avoidance of our feelings or indifference, but the ability to let go of what no longer serves our growth. Every time we feel that certain things no longer serve us and we are considering a new movement or path, the first step is to seek silence and tune in to our inner feelings and confront our fears, accepting them and then letting go of them after acknowledging the subconscious parts of ourselves that are trying to help us.

We need to have patience with ourselves when we are in a transitional period, and accept feeling insecure as a part of transcending to a new level of awareness. Frustration, confusion, sadness and anxiety are all normal when we are letting go of old patterns; they are signs of the shifts that are happening within us. Accept and acknowledge these feelings; it is perfect to express these feelings in physical movement or sounds. This will help the bottled-up emotions come out. My preferred mode of expression is a punching bag. You can scream, shout, hit a pillow with a baseball bat, run as hard as you can or do something creative like painting, drawing, dancing, singing or writing. Afterwards you can go back to silence and feel the energy flow and harmony in your body.

Another great way is with a partner; this is a technique called 'Haircut'. Decide with your partner how much time you will get to express your frustration, anger or grief (the average is three minutes). Then take three minutes to express it all: shout, scream or do whatever you feel like without physical contact with your partner. Your partner does not have to do anything; just be there. Afterwards, thank your partner and have a quiet moment to reflect.

Chakra 2 Disharmony

When chakra 2 is out of balance we will see more of: dependence on others (their approval, opinion, understanding), jealousy, suppression of feelings and denial, prejudice, excitability, taking everything personally, fixation on sex, addiction to drugs/eating/ nicotine/alcohol/vitamins/herbs/medicines. Other characteristics are: fanaticism, nostalgia, macho behaviour, possessiveness, being territorial, devotion, rigidity, obsession with structure and rules, admiration and fixation on celebrities or gurus/teachers, which can result in stalking.

- *Qualities to be developed:* courage, purity, self-sacrifice, surrender, honesty, tolerance, trust, letting go, flexibility, serenity, balance, common sense
- *Archetypes connected with chakra 2:* the victim, devotee, martyr, warrior, rebel (against convention)

Chakra 2 Overview

Element	Water
Physical	Adrenal glands, reproductive organs, colon, lower back, appendix, bladder
Consciousness	Enjoyment, expression of feelings, creativity, reproduction
Harmony	Honesty, truth, letting go, flexibility, serenity, hope
Disharmony	Denial, jealousy, guilt, dependency, blaming, suspicion
Sacred truth	Honour one another
Sacrament	Communion (holy union with the universal consciousness)
Energy content	Partnership (team spirit)

Fear	Fear of losing control
Special	Acceptance and acknowledgement of all feelings; to learn to interact consciously with others and form bonds with those who support our growth; letting go of toxic relationships
Emphasis	Competitive happiness, control
Affirmations	'I feel...' 'It is good for me...' 'I let go of...'

CASE STUDY: CHAKRA 2

I knew John very well; he and I had both been in martial arts for many years and we respected each other tremendously. He was a fifth-degree black belt and owned three schools of martial arts. In the martial arts field he was a leader and chair of several organizations. He was a tall man, in his late thirties, and looked like a bodybuilder. John came into my office quietly and, after saying hello, he sat down. Looking at his physiology I knew this was not going to be easy. He seemed to be depressed, and this appeared to be difficult for him. I soon understood why. John was 37 years old and one year into his second marriage with a fellow martial arts instructor. 'I can't do it anymore,' he whispered. 'There is no one else I can turn to!' I got an idea of what he was hinting at, but I needed to be sure. 'Are you talking about impotence?' He just nodded and stared at his feet, not saying a word. (By the way, this happened way before Viagra hit the market.) I started to dig deeper. What came out was that his first marriage had ended when he discovered that his wife had had an affair with one of his best friends. He had not talked to anyone about it and felt embarrassed. The most painful part of all of this was that he still saw his ex and his former close friend regularly at martial arts events and they seemed so happy. He had started to use marijuana to feel better, and also drank eight to 12 bottles of beer every day. His whole world had turned upside down; everyone looked up to him as the big hunk, the warrior, but he felt like a victim. He became very dependent on the opinion of others. He married one of his students who looked up to him; basically he had done it because he did not want to be alone. He was working out and exercising like crazy, and put a lot of emphasis on his physique. Criticism made him aggressive and he had been in a few fights. When he got high he'd mostly think about the past and how good it had been. I looked at him and said, 'John, you can get out of this if you really want to. It will take some work, but I am sure you can do it.' His eyes lit up: 'Do you really think I can go back to normal?'

'Yes, I believe so, but you cannot go back to the past and you have to stop escaping the present!'

Then I tested him using applied kinesiology. Unsurprisingly, chakra 2 seemed totally out of balance. Chakra 2 is about partnership, trust, letting go and accepting what is.

I gave John some serious homework to do, with two affirmations coupled with emotional balancing of the meridians of the colon (rigidity) and liver (forgiveness):

- ***General affirmation for balancing chakra 2*** (simultaneously massaging colon acupoints): 'I am flexible and accept and give lovingly, and am comfortable expressing my deepest feelings, now and continuously.'
- ***Personal affirmation for John*** (using liver acupoint): 'I accept and feel good about myself and let go of my past and forgive my ex-wife for cheating on me and accept her being with my friend, now and continuously.'

John was surprised that I could treat him with such simple statements. He was not impressed; he had expected some sort of pills or acupuncture for his problem. I explained to him that what he felt came from between his ears, and that what we were doing was correcting the problem at its source. I also explained to him that the power of emotional balance came from the combination of affirmations with acupressure. I said, 'When you do this six to eight times a day, it is as if you are getting a treatment from me six to eight times a day! So, I am saving you time and money by showing you how to do it yourself!' I explained to him that this therapy was the most powerful one available and that my success rate with phobias and emotional traumas was close to 97 per cent in all cases (this was not only true for my personal results but the accumulated average of all practitioners trained by me). 'This is cutting-edge preventive medicine I am prescribing for you; it is so advanced that it will take Western medicine decades to catch up with us!' He left feeling much better. I did not hear from him for seven weeks, when I ran into him at a martial arts event. 'How are you?' I asked. 'Could not be better,' he answered. He looked incredibly good, his face looked happy. 'How is "little John"?' I quipped. 'Working overtime to catch up!' he said in typically macho lingo. I knew he was his old self again. Later I spoke with him on the phone, when he called to thank me. After only five days his potency and libido had started to come back, and now he had more libido than during his first marriage and he was very happy.

CHAKRA 3 (*MANIPURA*): THE SOLAR PLEXUS

This is located in the area around the navel, the solar plexus. The consciousness is focused on self-responsibility and self-respect. Here we find survival intention, which warns of imminent danger and negativity coming from others and is the basis of self-esteem. To continue with the analogy of a growing baby: once it's fed and enjoying itself, the need will arise to discover its environment and explore the boundaries of the self. Connecting with others and learning about dangerous situations is needed for survival. The drive to explore is fire; fire is power and cleansing. This chakra controls metabolic processes and assimilation in the body. It keeps the balance between breaking down and regeneration. The fire element is needed to make the transformation from matter to energy. This chakra is the transitional chakra from a slow vibrational rate to faster vibrations that are tied into the subtle realms of love, intuition and expression. The associated physical organs are the stomach, small intestine, liver, gallbladder, kidneys, pancreas, spleen and middle spine.

Chakra 3 becomes disrupted by the misuse of will. This chakra deals with how we handle our life-force. It is all about the transformational use of our power to choose our life lessons and choose the directions that will sustain growth. Here most people get stuck in the comfort zone and their spiritual growth stagnates.

For some it is very difficult to distinguish between effortlessness (Level 3 consciousness) and being content. When we have all the material wealth we need to enjoy life to the fullest, what's next? You can now choose either to settle where you are or leave the material world and explore the unknown realms. We should live in charge of where we are going and not passively wait for events to react to.

One of the stumbling blocks is breaking free of ingrained thoughts that we have no creative power. Most of us have been adapting to others instead of carving our own paths. To harness the creative power of this chakra we have to choose to become the most influential force over all aspects of our lives. We have to find the inner power to create the outer movement, instead of responding to outer movement and suppressing ourselves. The idea here is to be able to respond to the outer world without losing touch with who we are and why we are here. When there is balance between our outer and inner reality, there is harmony in the solar plexus area. We should surrender to our inner reality without losing focus on where we are heading. For this we need to check on a regular basis with how we are doing inside.

Raising Chakra 3 Awareness

The blocks to overcome here are:

- Distrust of self: not being congruent with your inner feelings

- Getting stuck in your comfort zone and become passive or self-satisfied
- Not knowing what we really want, e.g. focusing on what you don't want
- Incongruence with your goals and desires
- Negative beliefs about ourselves (negative self-image)
- Buying into the myths, lies and negative beliefs of others (for example, feeling guilty about abundance or wealth)
- Over-humbleness, lack of assertiveness and self-pride
- Fear of the unknown, fear of change and rejection.

The third chakra demands that, in order for us to move to the next level, we should honour ourselves and keep connected with our inner feelings, and also respect the moment-to-moment survival information we receive from our intuition. The third chakra corresponds with the *emotional body* – the area through which emotions enter the body.

Chakra 3 Disharmony

When chakra 3 is out of balance, the most typical signs are lack of sympathy for others, becoming more selfish and detached, difficulty forgiving others, prejudice, harshness, criticism, keeping one's distance, intellectual pride and feeling superior, narrow-mindedness, being over-analytical and obsessed with details.

- **Qualities to be developed:** devotion, sympathy, love and having an open mind
- **Archetypes connected with chakra 3:** the lawyer, scientist, computer nerd, member of an analytical profession, surgeon, judge and teacher

Chakra 3 Overview

Element	Fire
Organs	Stomach, small intestine, liver, gallbladder, kidneys, pancreas, spleen and middle spine
Consciousness	Self-responsibility, honouring the self

Harmony	Forgiveness, being open to others, acknowledging inner feelings
Disharmony	Passivity, apathy, denial, judging, hopelessness, despair, prejudice, superiority, detachment
Sacred truth	Honour yourself
Sacrament	Confirmation (an expression of grace which enhances one's self-esteem and individuality)
Energy control	Personal power
Fears	Fear of not being worthy or loveable, fear of rejection
Special	Not to take external input too personally
Emphasis	Conditional love
Affirmations	'I can...' 'I am ready...' 'I am OK with rejection from others...'

CASE STUDY: CHAKRA 3

Ray was a 48-year-old judge, who came to see me because of a stomach ulcer.

His doctors told him that it was due to stress. He was now working part-time but was not very happy about it. His sister had raved about this doctor who used only herbs and natural methods, and urged him to come to see me. He was a robust man about six feet tall, and you could feel his authority. The way he sat with his back straight in the chair and the way he stared at me, oozed authority. I felt guilty of all the little crimes I had committed in my life. I tried to relax and question him. He did not answer easily; I had to pull everything out of him. When he did answer, he was completely detached as if he were a computer analyzing the situation and giving a status report. His wife, who accompanied him, was a petite blonde who was more aware of his emotional feelings. She told me later that lately he had changed a lot and had closed himself off emotionally. He did not want to socialize with many of their friends anymore because he thought they were boring.

After searching for 20 minutes for any clues she said, 'Everything changed after the "John Doe" case.' 'John Doe' was a lawyer who had committed fraud. He had been very well respected and Ray had met him socially several times, and sympathized with him. Ray had been asked to judge the case, but refused for personal reasons. 'John Doe' was found guilty on many counts: money-laundering, tax fraud and more. After that Ray had gradually changed and had become literally sick to his stomach.

Tests revealed severe disharmony of the third chakra; this normally can result in digestive problems including ulcers, disorders of the pancreas and low blood sugar. When I then questioned Ray, based on this diagnosis, he indeed had symptoms of low blood sugar and digestive problems, which were confirmed by laboratory tests. What I found out was that when Ray was young, he had had a close friend in whom he confided and to whom he told everything. He knew that he could not trust his friend, but because it was difficult for him to make social contact, he went against his feelings. His friend betrayed his trust by telling his parents about an accident that had happened and about which Ray had been afraid to tell his parents. 'John Doe' in some way reminded him of his friend and the incident had triggered old feelings. He suppressed those feelings and never shared them with anyone! Actually it came down to the fact that Ray thought subconsciously he did not deserve to be a judge because he could not even trust himself.

Chakra 3, when in disharmony, will allow our negative beliefs about ourselves to go rampant: we then start buying into the lies and negative beliefs of others. We no longer can depend on our own judgement. It was tough to convince Ray that I preferred to work first only with affirmations once I had a clear diagnosis of an imbalanced chakra. I also make use of bio-energetic remedies. He was not convinced, but decided to give it a chance for four weeks and then we would evaluate.

- **General affirmation for balancing chakra 3** (simultaneously massaging the pancreas/spleen acupoints): 'I honour myself and I can easily connect with others and appreciate their opinions and feelings, while staying connected with myself, now and continuously.'
- **Personal affirmation for Ray:** 'I accept and love myself and let go of my anxiety, my worries and self-judgement, now and continuously.'

After four weeks Ray came back alone; he was a changed person. Just one week after his visit he had quit taking his stomach medication and had resumed his work full-time. He not only felt much better, but he had also started up an old hobby again: painting. He had also visited 'John Doe' in prison and had felt better after talking with him and felt he understood him. He was very excited and also apologetic for not trusting my methods. I was especially impressed with the complete change in his physiology. 'This stuff really works!' I heard myself thinking.

CHAKRA 4 (*ANAHATA*): HEART CHAKRA

This is located in the chest cavity. The consciousness here is focused on love, harmony and nurturing compassion for ourselves and our actions in the world.

To continue with the analogy of a growing baby, once it is fed, enjoying itself and exploring the outside world and other people, it will start bonding with other children. Affinity will lead to the development of loving friendships and relationships.

The elements here are air or a combination of water and fire. Here we find lessons about love, commitment, forgiveness, compassion, harmony and anger, resentment, abandonment, grief, bitterness, loneliness, regret, sorrow, co-dependency and self-centredness.

Many people believe that the heart is the centre for unconditional love; that is not true. Unconditional love is the highest virtue and will be at the level of the seventh chakra. The heart wants to be loved; it wants to give love but in return it wants to receive it back. That is the reason why so many people are heartbroken: they give love with the expectation that everything is going to be fine forever after. That is not the case in real life: there are many bumps, detours and roadblocks to overcome, and these are essential for our growth process. For that reason commitment and also marriage are essential to growth. Only when there is commitment and a clear goal for spiritual growth will we make it over the bumps and grow exponentially. Holding on to negative emotions from the past, whether they are directed toward others or ourselves, or intentionally causing pain to others, will deplete life-force from the body.

Fear is one of the disruptive forces of the loving harmony of the heart. Hostility is the other disruptive energy. Tapping into the energy of love reduces fears such as the fear of commitment, loneliness, being betrayed and being vulnerable. The potential of this chakra is in direct relation to the degree to which we love ourselves; this will enable us to be more receptive to receiving and giving love and warmth. Lack of self-worth is detrimental to our existence and will cause us to develop negative beliefs such as worthlessness and being unlovable. Building our self-esteem and capacity for intimacy is very important for spiritual growth.

The energy pulsating from this chakra will direct us to evaluate our beliefs and integrity. By accepting anyone or anything lacking integrity, we pollute our spirit and body. It will require awareness to re-educate ourselves and focus on how we short-change ourselves on love, and how to change that.

Raising Chakra 4 Awareness

The fourth chakra is exactly in the middle of the upper and lower chakras. It is the pivotal chakra because it's the beginning of the higher vibrations which correspond with the higher level of consciousness. It is the transformational bridge from body to spirit. When there is no connection between the lower and higher chakras we choose to focus on either the physical or the ethereal. Something very common is that many so-called spiritual people detach completely from their bodies and focus entirely on the spirit. The most powerful moving force of the heart chakra is pure love. This is the essence of human nature: being able to receive and give love. Loving others really means accepting and cherishing them for who they are. It does not mean you get to decide whether or not they need changing. It is not up to you to force them but to support them even if you believe they could make better choices. The basis for this is to have open and honest communication. Love is a commitment, and *not* a natural process; our nature is to run away from confrontation, not to look for it. Love is challenging and it requires a strong third chakra (honouring yourself) and knowing your limitations and how far you are prepared to go. Not knowing your boundaries or not honouring yourself will result in losing your identity and giving up your happiness. The heart is the centre of forgiveness; nurturing our power to forgive and using it as much as possible (you cannot forgive too much), without losing sight of ourselves, is the best way to keep the heart open and in harmony. Spiritual growth is the process of becoming aware of our creative powers and the gradual increase of awareness of our inner beauty and to be able to become a channel for expressing God's love in the form of love, joy, harmony and peace. This can only happen if we are willing and are able to open our hearts.

Chakra 4 Disharmony

When chakra 4 is out of balance, the most typical signs are attachment, anger, greed, egoism, lack of assertiveness, over-protectiveness of the self, daydreaming, lack of objectivity, always searching for the better and more beautiful, thinking that looks are more important than content, emotional instability, doubt and mood swings.

- **Qualities to be developed:** self-esteem, serenity, self-control, purity, altruism, greater balance, precision

- *Archetypes connected with chakra 4:* the artist, negotiator, painter and actor

Chakra 4 Overview

Elements	Air (Fire and Water)
Organs	Lungs, heart, thymus
Consciousness	Love, compassion, joy
Harmony	Understanding, happiness, self-acceptance, having a reason to live
Disharmony	Regret, dependency, sadness, grief, trying to fulfil someone else's expectations, indifference, abandonment
Sacred truth	Love is divine power
Sacrament	Marriage (honours the essential need to love and take care of oneself so that one can fully love another)
Energy content	Emotional power
Fears	Fear of commitment, betrayal, loneliness, fear of being vulnerable, fear of following your heart
Special	To accept loved ones the way they are without trying to change them
Emphasis	To work on unconditional love
Affirmations	'I love _____ the way he/she is...' 'I am worthy to receive love.' 'I deserve...'

CASE STUDY: CHAKRA 4

Sandra looked at me with her big blue eyes, waiting for my reaction. She had just told me that she had been a prostitute six years ago; she was accustomed to seeing shock, disgust or some other sign of rejection at this news. I'd met her about two years previously when she'd started coming to my workshops. She was studying to become a health practitioner. I waited for a second before giving an answer. I was not shocked at all;

I'd always felt a strange energy around her and it was as if she did not belong in the group of people studying alternative medicine. Now I could place that energy and a lot of things made more sense: the way she dressed to hide her femininity and how she was always very quiet and visibly uncomfortable in the group of therapists. She had no friends that I knew of. 'I have a friend who also used to be a prostitute,' I said. 'I think the two of you should meet; she is now studying to become a massage therapist and maybe you can support one another.' She looked relieved that I did not judge or condemn her as many whom she had trusted had done.

Sandra had come to see me because of her 'asthma'; she had been using an inhaler and all sorts of chemical drugs, but lately it was getting worse. She was advised to give away her two cats and her dog. She had allergies to house-dust, milk, pollen, perfume, antibiotics, cats, dogs and birds. Doing a series of tests to find any underlying cause for her asthma (she had had this for eight years and had had to stop her prostitution work because of it), to my surprise at the time the most prominent weakness in her energetic body was her heart chakra. After exploring that further with additional questions, she admitted to having been sexually molested by an uncle who had lived with them when she was young. It had all started when she was five years old and had lasted for seven years. After that she was raped twice when she was 17 years old. When she was 19, a boyfriend forced her into prostitution. So it was not strange at all that she had quite a lot of anger toward men; she was now in a lesbian relationship and said she felt happy and secure, but was afraid to tell her mum. Her partner was an older woman almost her mother's age.

Hostility is detrimental to the heart chakra; being unforgiving only adds fuel to the fire. This, in Sandra's case, was coupled with a lack of self-worth and feelings of unworthiness that were constantly reinforced by her being judged by others. She had become a chain smoker and also drank a good deal of wine (a bottle or a bottle and a half a day). She also told me that she had initially wanted to become a dancer or actress, but had given up those dreams long ago because of the non-supportive environment she'd grown up in.

I told her that her asthma was psychosomatic, as were her allergies. 'You have asthma and you have allergies; both have the same cause. You don't have asthma because of your allergies, as many doctors told you.' I further explained that her allergies were a way of rejecting all the things she did not think she was worthy of having: the house-dust allergy indicated that she did not feel she deserved to have the nice house she was living in, the milk allergy indicated a symbolic rejection of her mother (because she expected her mother to reject her), the pollen allergy was because she rejected flowers which symbolized romantic attention from men. The perfume allergy was her rejecting herself (as a prostitute she used perfume a lot to cleanse herself emotionally of men) and the allergy to antibiotics indicated that her life was not worth saving. She loved her cats and dog, but she subconsciously did not believe she deserved them. Birds were symbolic of pigeons or doves, and therefore of love and peace, which she also felt she did not deserve. I said to her, 'If my professor from medical school could hear me speak today, he would kill himself, but this is what my tests indicate; actually it is all good news. If you love yourself, there is a reasonable chance that all of your symptoms will disappear!'

Sandra was very happy with my diagnosis and prognosis and could not wait to start with her therapy. I gave her the following two affirmations to do every day, eight to 10 times a day for six weeks. She also got some homeopathic and herbal medicine to assist her body in cleansing itself.

- *General affirmation for balancing chakra 4*
  (simultaneously massaging the lung points): 'I love and respect myself deeply and I am worthy to receive plenty of love and forgive easily all those who hurt me, now and continuously.'

● ***Personal affirmation for Sandra:*** 'I accept and love
myself just the way I am with my past and forgive
myself for everything I have attracted in my life.'

After six weeks I saw Sandra again; she had stopped using the
inhaler and had quit smoking two weeks after she'd started
the affirmations. She had an occasional bout of asthma, but
always knew why and would then work to let go of those
feelings. She had decided to tell her mother everything and
was anxious about it. I told her to continue the affirmations
until she was completely symptom-free. Two months later
we met at a seminar and she told me she had not had any
symptoms for three weeks. Her mother had been very
supportive when she'd come out to her, which had also taken
place three weeks before. What a coincidence!

CHAKRA 5 (*VISHUDDHA*): THROAT CHAKRA

This is located in the neck region at the base of the throat and is
associated with the ability to communicate or express our creativity
and inner self, thereby allowing a sense of connection with the
world and ourselves. This consciousness is an expression of our
inner self to manifest ourselves in the world.

In our analogy of the exploring child, after bonding, the
necessity will grow in the child to express its most intimate feelings
and to be clear and truthful about its boundaries and identity.

The elements associated with the fifth chakra are sound and
ether. Ether is the binding element of water, air and fire. Ether
represents the ultrafine magnetic force field.

The fifth chakra acts as a focal point for the heart energy of
the fourth chakra and the mind energy of the sixth chakra. Its
energy is formed by the willpower to choose for self-expression
and the truth. Every area of our lives, especially illness and health,
is directly affected by the karma we generate by our choices and
how we arrive at making those choices. Clarity and wisdom are
the basis of true authority and the direct result of the truth of the
sixth chakra in harmony with the loving power of the heart chakra.

Every choice we make is the result of the equilibrium between our emotional and mental state (right and left brain). If there is a struggle between these states, there will be disharmony in the throat chakra. Prolonged disharmony can result in physical ailments of the throat, thyroid, mouth, jaws, teeth, gums, parathyroid, trachea, neck and hypothalamus.

Chakra 5 is the centre where the energy of the vibrations in our body intermingles and takes form. By expressing our inner world we channel unwanted or disharmonious energies out and harmonize ourselves with our environment. By doing this we can shape our environment and harmonize this as well. By harmonizing our emotions, thoughts, feelings and intuition with the outside world, we can constantly monitor the effect of our expression and the response we get from our environment. This way we get an exchange on many levels simultaneously by combining the input of what we see, hear, feel and sense.

Raising Chakra 5 Awareness

Communication is the exchange of information. Interestingly enough, a person can manipulate the words he uses through intonation and timbre, but he can never completely manipulate the non-verbal parts of communication. Our antenna will always pick up stress, distrust and lies, even if we are not consciously aware of this. Communication also helps to structure our thoughts and feelings and helps us to create clarity. To communicate efficiently, the receiver must check if she has understood the message and the sender should check if the other really got the message. When we are having an inner dialogue, the communication becomes blurry and ineffective and will, in most cases, lead to misunderstanding. When we notice that the other person is not giving us appropriate attention and we keep on talking, we are stuck in a dysfunctional pattern. Congruent communication is when the non-verbal and verbal signals we are sending convey the same message. When chakra 5 is in balance there is clarity, patience, justice, dignity, understanding, insight, devotion and prudence, and our message is well articulated.

When we express ourselves truthfully, we fine-tune our inner harmonics and relieve stressors. By not expressing ourselves truthfully, we create more tension in our body and we lose energy. The other downside of not honouring the truth is that we harm ourselves and also, on an etheric level, others will sense our tension and disharmony as well. Neale D. Walsch, bestselling author of the *Conversations with God* series, writes in one of his newsletters the following: 'By honest self-expression, we do not give ourselves away.' Most people give in here, compromise there, adapt there and swallow the truth a little bit not to hurt others. It is very subtle; it never seems like a big deal or hurtful to anyone. One day you wake up and you discover that you are not the person you thought you were. You've stopped going to dance class because it was inconvenient, you don't read anymore but watch videos, you've stopped going to the gym due to lack of time. Actually you've given up being the Magnificent Joyful Exploring You and have become the amiable overweight lazy person most of your friends sympathize with. Somewhere deep inside you still yearn for the inner truth and integrity of your youth, for that person who would never have compromised just to keep the game going.

This is exactly what a balanced fifth chakra would never let happen. We have to keep finding ways to express ourselves joyfully to show our gratitude. Dancing, painting, walking, making music, writing poems, making art are all part of our self-expressing creativity. If we forget who we are, we malnourish ourselves and stop our development, and sooner or later we lose the joy, excitement, tenderness and warmth that we all have in us.

Chakra 5 Disharmony

When chakra 5 is out of balance, the most typical results are isolation, withholding information, twisting the truth, absentmindedness, focus on the self, always being busy, preoccupation with details, manipulativeness, setting people at one another's throats.

- **Qualities to be developed:** tolerance, devotion, accuracy and sympathy

- ***Archetypes connected with chakra 5:*** the technician, project manager, superior, manager, coach

Chakra 5 Overview

Elements	Sound and Ether
Organs	Throat, thyroid, neck, shoulder, oesophagus, mouth, jaws, teeth, gums, parathyroid, trachea, hypothalamus
Consciousness	Expressing inner feelings, creativity, inner truth, communication with others
Harmony	Respect and openness, adult communication
Disharmony	Withdrawal, punishment, suppressing emotions
Sacred truth	Surrender personal will to Divine will
Sacrament	Confession (cleansing one's spirit of negative acts of will)
Energy content	The power of will
Fear	Fear of hurting someone else
Special	To stay honest even when it is painful
Emphasis	To find different ways to express your creativity
Affirmations	'I speak...' 'It is good for others and for me to...' 'It is healthy for me...'

CASE STUDY: CHAKRA 5

Looking through my files to find a suitable case to share with you for chakra 5, I found many more cases than for the other chakras. I think there are so many cases of chakra 5 problems because we are all too willing to compromise and not be completely honest in our communication. We think we do not want to hurt others' feelings but in reality we are afraid of being rejected for what we are saying, so we compromise on our feelings and cause stress in chakra 5. Another reason is that we are not always congruent with what we say. This is easily measurable and recognizable as stress patterns in a voice analysis. Every time we say something that is not true or only partially true, we stress our fifth chakra.

I was at a party hosted by Simon, a friend of mine. It was busy and there were many friends, colleagues and business associates there. Walter came up to me and asked, 'Roy, do you have a minute?' I knew something was wrong with him; he'd broken into a cold sweat and his face was pale, his pupils small. We went into a room that my friend used as a home-office. Walter was a well-to-do manager of a medium-sized company; he looked younger than his 52 years. I knew him also from my workshops and I enjoyed his sense of humour and his enthusiasm for emotional balance.

He told me he had experienced a sudden sharp pain in his sinuses. He did not know what to; he thought he could go to his GP to get painkillers, but had decided to check with me first. I performed a quick check-up on him with muscle-testing. What emerged, to my surprise, was that he had a blockage of his throat chakra. After some searching, we found the reason for this: he was upset with our mutual friend, Simon, who had promised to include him in a joint venture he had been setting up a few months earlier. Walter had not heard anymore about the deal and had thought everything was on hold. At the party, though, he'd found out that the joint venture was up and running and already successful without him. He was very angry. Just after hearing this, he'd turned round to go to the loo and encountered Simon. Simon had asked how he was doing and automatically he'd answered in his usual way: 'Great, what a great party.' After 15 minutes he got the pain.

I started to treat him right away, and after 10 minutes his pain was completely gone. He was amazed. Then I started to talk to him to find out what he was doing generally that might be stressing chakra 5. What we found was that he

101

regularly had throat infections and was very protective of his throat and always wore a scarf, even in summer. He had also been diagnosed with hypothyroidism and was taking synthetic thyroid hormones for that. Last but not least, he had recurrent neck and shoulder pain. I told him that his symptoms indicated chronic stress of the throat chakra and that I suspected he had a problem with being completely honest to others. He said, 'That's not completely true!' Then he started to laugh, and added, 'I guess you are right,' then our eyes met and he started to laugh again because he had just told another lie. 'OK, I admit it. I sometimes have a problem saying what I really think!' '*Sometimes?*' I asked and looked at him again. He looked down and became visibly uncomfortable, and my impression was that for the first time he was really trying to say what he felt: 'Actually, you are right. I never say what I really mean!' He let out a sigh and continued to look down, completely lost in his thoughts. I explained to him that I completely sympathized with him and that this was an issue I'd struggled with for many years. 'I will help you if you are committed to telling the truth!' He agreed and I gave him the following affirmation to do at home for the next six to eight weeks, at least six times a day, while massaging the acupoints indicated.

- **General affirmation for balancing chakra 5**
  (simultaneously massaging the Triple Burner acupoint): 'I express my thoughts and feelings honestly and I am truthful to myself and others, now and continuously.'

When we started practising this, Walter could not finish the sentence without stumbling; after the first four tries, though, it came out with ease.

Walter and I met two weeks later, when I was doing an evening lecture. During the break he came up to me to thank me. 'It is miraculous how good I feel,' he said. 'And you know the best part? It is easier than I expected!' He told me how his relationship with his wife had improved now that he expressed his emotions; also at work the whole atmosphere was much better. I wished for a brief moment that all cases could be this simple. My experience, after working with the emotional balance technique for five years now, is that it makes everything easier and it speeds up healing of any chronic disease.

May this case illustrate how important it is to stay true to ourselves and to honour our inner feelings and express our thoughts.

CHAKRA 6 (*AJNA*): BROW CHAKRA

This is located between the eyebrows and is connected with our intuition, or Third Eye, which allows us to express and validate our dreams and/or imagination.

The endocrine gland connected to the sixth chakra is the pituitary. This is the last chakra within the physical body and is most known for its spiritual qualities and use in spiritual practice.

The consciousness here is the expression of our insights, intuition and connection with universal love. When the sixth chakra is strong we can start to see energy and vibrations and move toward clairvoyance. Basically it comes down to connecting with the universe and experiencing unconditional love. The fifth chakra, according to Carolyn Myss, is about progressing through the maturation of will from the perception that everyone and everything around you has authority over you, through the perception that you alone have authority over you, to the final perception (chakra 6) that the authority comes from aligning yourself to God's will. The sixth chakra helps us to align with the reason why we have incarnated in this world. We come here to experience first-hand how to deal with certain situations and, as soon as the lesson is learned, we can let go of the patterns needed to create those situations. The sixth chakra and the fifth chakra allow us to return to our inner core and stay focused on our path. Our ultimate goal is to resolve our old issues and move on.

This chakra also helps us to attract the situations needed to continue to evolve spiritually. We can observe with more clarity and see what really is going on; we also get more efficient at creating visual images. The lack of clarity that most of us experience is the result of our projection of the past onto our current reality. We will then react as if still in the old situation. By not letting go of our conditioned patterns, we keep recreating our past without making any progress.

The most important step in spiritual growth is to become a neutral observer; we can then observe ourselves without prejudice and take decisions based on what the best outcome will be for the spiritual growth of all involved. In collaboration with the seventh chakra, we get inspired and connect with higher sources of knowledge and this energy can manifest in our loves. The Brow Chakra is also where we manifest our intellectual mind within the wider context of the spiritual mind. We create bad karma by using our intellectual mind to dissociate from our feelings or to forge destructive creations that harm humanity or planet Earth.

Raising Chakra 6 Awareness

The intuitive mind is the spiritual mind, and is the basis for inspiration and new creations. By focusing and emphasizing the logical, analytical mind, we suppress the spiritual mind. Most people are afraid of silence because they are then confronted by all the chatter in their minds. Turning the TV, radio or music on is not the solution. We should not silence the mind, but let it quiet down by speaking out. This is where the power of meditation comes in. Meditating helps us to calm our mind; then we can connect to the source of our thoughts. This is referred to as *the gap* and is the moment of silence in which we create or access the next thought. That moment of silence is the moment of infinite new possibilities. Everything is possible and we get a glimpse of infinity and eternity. This is how we keep connected with our spirit. Our spirit does all the work: gathering information, getting people into our lives. By going into *the gap* we can effortlessly access this information. *Silence is where all the answers are.* Practising visualization will develop our creative powers.

The choices we make are the karmic fuel for our spiritual growth. When we experience problems with letting go of the past, this is expressed as grief. Grief is stagnation and the slowing down of our vibrations. By acknowledging grief and letting it express itself, we create movement: if we don't, we risk depression.

Chakra 6 Disharmony
When chakra 6 is out of balance, the most typical signs are: manifestation of the ego with possessiveness, attachment, anger, feeling hurt, dishonesty and, as a result, indifference ('most people are boring') and an obsession with accumulating knowledge. Also possible negativity, feelings of inferiority, self-pity, depression, feeling unhappy with own performance or success.

- *Qualities to be developed:* unconditional love, compassion, letting go of being driven by the ego, altruism
- *Archetypes connected with chakra 6:* the charismatic leader, philosopher, philanthropist, visionary, peacemaker

Chakra 6 Overview

Element	Light
Organs	Pituitary, eyes, sinus
Consciousness	Connecting with universal truth (omniscience)
Harmony	Trusting our intuition, following our insights, acknowledging our universal love, taking time to meditate
Disharmony	Attachment, greed, dishonesty, dissociation with our feelings and intuition, not creating time for silence
Sacred truth	Seek only the truth
Sacrament	Ordination (recognizes the unique insight and wisdom that lead one to helping others; making sacred one's path of service)

Energy content	The power of the mind
Fear	Fear of total surrender
Special	Connecting with *the gap*
Emphasis	To learn about unconditional happiness
Affirmations	'I know...' 'I understand...' 'It is possible for me...'

CASE STUDY: CHAKRA 6

Susan was not happy at all. She actually was very upset. She was a journalist for a well-known magazine and had interviewed me just one week previously. She had told me then of her recurrent headaches and sinusitis, and I had offered my help. She was a nervous woman in her early forties and she was a chain smoker. She was a fast talker and very uncomfortable with silence. She loved to make jokes and was especially good at creating humour about herself. The reason she was upset was that I had just told her that her headaches were her way of escaping responsibility and getting attention. She started to tell me that she did not care for attention and that she was fed up with people telling her that she was not able to get in touch with her emotions. I had not referred to her emotions yet, so she must have guessed that I was going to say that. I let her talk. I wanted to tell her there was a lot of anger inside of her, when she said, 'I know you think that I have a lot of anger inside, but what do you expect?' It took me a few minutes to realize that she could catch my thoughts even before I finished them.

I had tested her and found the problem was a totally disturbed chakra 6. I'd just wanted to ask her about her youth when she'd started talking about how she'd grown up in Indonesia and that she'd never felt comfortable around people, because she could see 'things'. She also could see light around people. All of this had disappeared when she'd seen in a dream that her mother was going to die in a car accident. She was seven at the time; the next morning she told her mother to stay home, but her mother laughed at her and told her not to be silly. Her mother died that same day. Shortly after that the whole family had moved to the Netherlands and she had shut herself off from receiving any more psychic messages. She had been suffering from headaches ever since.

I explained to Susan that she had a very sensitive chakra 6; by not acknowledging her intuition she was creating her physical complaints. I also explained that this was why she had problems dealing with silence and was always either talking or listening to music. By smoking so much she was suppressing her emotions. Focusing on others instead of herself had led her to become a journalist; this way she would never be the one getting the attention. The reason she had problems with relationships was that she would get possessive, attached and clingy; she would feel anxiety and fear and in the end her partner could no longer deal with it and would leave.

She was perplexed by my diagnosis: 'How do you know all of that?' she asked. 'I used the same chakra 6 to pick up this information,' I said. 'You can do the same when you are quiet.' She started to tell me how, often, during an interview, she knew things, and how she could never explain to her subjects why she'd asked certain questions. I told her that she could balance herself and benefit even more by listening to this inner voice and trusting it. 'If you do, you will find more peace and happiness,' I said. Here is the affirmation that I gave her to do over the next four weeks:

- **General affirmation for balancing chakra 6**
  (simultaneously massaging the Conception Vessel acupoint): 'I fully trust my intuition and insights and accept my omniscience and love myself for who I am, now and continuously.'

I also advised Susan to take a class on primordial sound meditation, a mantra meditation system brought to the West by Deepak Chopra. Four weeks later she came to show me an article she had written on meditation. She was doing much better, felt calm inside and had found some new friends in her meditation group. Her headaches were almost gone, and though her sinuses were still a nuisance, they were much better than they had been. When I spoke with her some three months later she was a totally different person; she had quit smoking and stopped all the medications she'd been taking for her sinuses and headaches. Once in a while she would feel something and know exactly what she was suppressing. She was very happy and looked five years younger.

CHAKRA 7 (*SAHASRARA*): CROWN CHAKRA

This is located at the top of the head and is connected to Universal Energy. This chakra is a holographic projection into space and is not in the actual physical body. It is a transformational point to the astral dimension (out-of-body dimension). The seventh chakra is the ultimate synergy of intent and creation. It is the creator and destroyer of matter and it directly influences the anti-matter, the blueprint of creation. It relates to values, courage, natural leadership, humanitarianism, total honesty, the power to influence matter, the capacity to explain complex spiritual material and remain non-judgemental and compassionate, and the ability to see the big picture. It is the chakra of inspiration, spirituality and devotion, and the indestructible ability to trust life.

The crown chakra teaches how to stay in the moment. Most of us are tied to the past; by forgiving others, ourselves and giving empowering meanings to what we used to consider our traumas, we let go of the hurts and unresolved emotions. We learn how to change and understand energy, how to surrender and trust, how to be inspired and commit to our life's mission. By consciously judging our thinking processes, we no longer give energy to cyclical patterns and we expand our self-imposed boundaries. The crown chakra keeps us focused on our responsibility and alerts us when we hand it over to others. The seventh chakra allows us to break free from the karma laid upon us through our parents, education, social and cultural conditioning, and our geographical location.

By connecting with the spirit, we can see wrongdoing even if we have been raised to consider it normal. We can see what is wrong with certain customs and habits in our family or culture. We do not need any outside knowledge for that, it is already in us; we just have to allow it to flow through us. The dogmas of religion can be accepted for what they are and we can connect to the Source directly.

When we neglect or ignore our true self, we will get repeated warnings and signals that will grow stronger through time. We will, sooner or later, be confronted in a way that will be difficult to ignore. Using the power of chakra 7, we can release negative beliefs and replace them with empowering visualizations and affirmations. We should be alert to any disempowering belief we have overlooked.

Raising Chakra 7 Awareness

The dualism between surrender and creation at the level of chakra 7 means we move in effortless manifestation. This is called *Siddhi* consciousness. The *Siddhi* consciousness is the state of awareness where there is absolutely no doubt and no delay between the creative intent and its materialization into matter. It is the ultimate state of being in which we create effortlessly and instantly. This is because this level of consciousness does not create its effects through the mind; it works through anti-matter. The mind often is the biggest barrier to experiencing this level of consciousness, which is linked to unconditional happiness. It is in chakra 7 where the awareness is of the perfect state; where there is inner knowing and you align yourself graciously with universal energy. Through silence and spiritual practice, we can access more and more of the *Siddhi* consciousness. The *Siddhi* consciousness relates to the state of 'pure joy' (*amanda*). We experience some of it on occasion when we sit and watch the sun come up, or see a rainbow or hold a newborn baby in our arms. In those moments we dip into the 'pure joy' that is always there in our seventh chakra.

To develop and grow spiritually we should never skip the basics and should take care of our body and our basic needs. Nurture your body and yourself, so you won't be distracted in your spiritual practice. It is not correct to believe that in order to grow spiritually we should give up all material things and conduct a life of austerity. That would only be helpful if we had become attached and were stuck in a comfort zone.

Chakra 7 Disharmony

When chakra 7 is out of balance, the most typical signs are: pride, ambition, arrogance, power games, depression, aloofness, irritation, impatience, withdrawal, isolation, a need to control everything, harshness, insomnia, confusion.

- **Qualities to be developed:** softness, sympathy, caring for others, patience, learning to be vulnerable when you are a leader
- **Archetypes connected with chakra 7:** the general, government official, leader, chairman, CEO, conqueror

Chakra 7 Overview

Element	Thought
Organ	Pineal gland
Consciousness	*Siddhi* consciousness: flow state, unconditional happiness, effortlessness
Harmony	Truth, compassion, unconditional love, forgiveness
Disharmony	Attachment to past or future, dishonesty, indifference, hatred, extroversion, hostility
Sacred truth	Live in the present moment
Sacrament	Extreme unction (the grace to finish unfinished business daily, thus allowing a person to live in the present)
Energy content	Our spiritual connector
Fear	Loss of focus
Special	Synchronicity: meaningful meditative practice is essential if we are to connect

Emphasis	To leave the details of manifestation to the universe
Affirmations	'I am...' 'I am in balance now and continuously...' 'I create...' 'I manifest...'

CASE STUDY: CHAKRA 7

I was attending a seminar to become a certified Fire-walk Instructor, given by one of the originators of the fire-walking movement in the US, Peggy Dylan. This took place in Switzerland. I was very impressed with Peggy; she was one of the most sincere and spiritual people I had met in a long time. Her incredible connection with the powers of the universe became apparent every day when we were outside and eagles would appear as soon as she started to meditate. During this seminar, one of the participants, Therese, got completely confused after a session about rebirthing. This is a special breathing technique that brings you in contact with your deepest emotional traumas. She looked a little bit disorientated and was repeating over and over: 'I don't want to die, I don't want to die!'

I tested her and the only thing that I could find was disharmony in chakra 7. This probably came about when she had experienced some memories of previous lives. Later she told me that she was an Egyptian high priest who'd died violently at the hands of an opposing sect many centuries ago. She was also someone who had been practising meditation for years and had been on the spiritual path for the last 20 years. She was a very loving and kind person and very charismatic. Therese conducted seminars on feminine spirituality all over Europe.

I worked on her chakra 7, massaging acupoints and focusing my mind on synchronizing her energies. After 15 minutes she calmed down and her eyes returned to normal again. She thanked me for the help and told me that she was out of her body all that time, but was reliving what she believed to be the past and just could not let go of the agony. She said that my energy was very calming and helped her to come back to this reality. She told me that she sometimes suffered from depression, especially in wintertime (which is a weakness of the pineal gland, which is tied to chakra 7). She also went through periods when she did not want to be with people and would withdraw into the woods for three to four weeks at a time, just meditating. This is the affirmation I gave her:

- *General affirmation for balancing chakra 7*
  (simultaneously massaging the Governor and
  Conception Vessel acupoints): 'I am fully connected
  with Divinity and unconditional love and I am
  completely balanced on all levels of my being, now
  and continuously.'

We stayed in touch and Therese has not experienced any depression or other symptoms since.

It is rare to find disturbances only in chakra 7.

SUMMARY

This chapter has given you a very in-depth look at the chakras, with many new insights that I have been able to present after working for years with these gateways. As a clinician I can state that due to this knowledge, my ability to support healing in those who seek my help has increased exponentially. By combining the tremendous powers of the chakras to help change limiting patterns with the ancient knowledge of acupuncture, a complete new science and therapy has been born, unparalleled in alternative medicine as far as I know. Although this book has no intention of replacing professional health care, it may alleviate the suffering of millions of people while helping them to gain insights that will ease them on their spiritual path. The more than 1,000 doctors and therapists trained in these techniques have experienced the same excellent results as I: more than 95 per cent success in treating phobias, post-traumatic stress and more.

Later on in this book I will refer back to the specific affirmations for each chakra so you can use them to access your unlimited potential. Some of you may already have recognized areas that will require work. By carefully reading this chapter you will gain insights into your personality. More than one chakra may need treatment. You can select to treat them one by one, or all simultaneously. Every time you focus on one affirmation you are connecting to the related chakra and will help to harmonize it and support your healing and health intelligence.

Also, the seven case studies are meant to help you find the tools you need. The good news is: you cannot go wrong with these affirmations. You cannot 'overdose' or 'over-treat' yourself. These are just positive messages you are sending to your brain.

While doing the affirmations it is best to massage the indicated acupoint (which you will find described in Part II). This will make all the difference. When people first use affirmations they can meet a lot of resistance from the negative programming in their subconscious mind. When we massage the acupoints, we keep the energy flowing and harmonize the body with the message (affirmation). That is the secret of emotional balance.

You can start with your preferred affirmations right now, either one after another or spaced in time, or just choose one to repeat two times a day or more. Everything you do will assist you in your progress.

The Only Time that Exists Is Now

The most logical way to work with more than one chakra is to start with the one lowest in vibration, and then move higher up. So normally we would start with the root chakra followed by the sacral chakra, the solar plexus chakra, etc. Because you cannot go wrong you don't have to worry if you have all or just one of the signs and symptoms associated with a given chakra. You may recognize aspects of yourself in all seven. That's fine; just commit to work on this for at least four weeks and you will find significant changes in your patterns and the way you look at the world and how you feel on the inside. This work can be combined with any existing therapy, meditation or spiritual practice.

CHAPTER 7

CELL-MEMORY: UNLIMITED GIGABYTES OF KARMIC INFORMATION

BURNING NEGATIVE MEMORY (KARMA)

We are living in an 'information age'; the ones in control of this information are all billionaires. The flow of information has increased within a short span of time. Computers get faster, with greater capacity. There is no end in sight.

Despite all this advanced technology, however, computers are nowhere near reaching the information packed in a single human cell. This cell is so small that we need a microscope to get a glimpse of its structure. It is a powerhouse packed with more information than we can grasp. Each tiny little cell is a holographic representation of the whole body. The science of cloning is based on this idea. Most of this information is not yet accessible to us. We are learning more and more about this microscopic universe day by day. For those who believe in reincarnation, I will offer some interesting insights into how we can access some of this information. For those who do not believe, I will demonstrate how the past still comes to haunt us through our ancestors and how we still have to deal with their karma whether we like it or not. This chapter is crucial because it is the foundation to the way in which emotional balance and some other techniques help us to let go of the past and to burn negative karma faster than you can read this chapter.

CELL-MEMORY: YOUR MINI-HOLOGRAM

The information I am about to disclose may change the way you deal with your life forever. Ask anyone about cell-memory and they will either give you a blank stare or start talking about how many gigabytes their computer has. Some may even think you are talking about the latest cell-phone with memory. Cell-memory, though, is the information that is present in any one of your body's cells. If we were to reproduce you by cloning one of your cells, we would get an exact replica with the same memories, scars and thoughts as the original. Isn't it interesting that a hologram of you can be constructed from the information in your cells? In other words, a cell can store incoming information similarly to the way a computer saves onto a CD or DVD.

YOUR ANCESTORS LIVE ON IN YOUR CELLS

Besides our own information, the cells also carry information about the unresolved issues and suppressed emotions of previous generations. Lucky for us part of this information gets 'bumped' by similar information with a stronger signal. Also, after some generations the information starts to fade away unless the behavioural pattern responsible for creating the information is also passed on and repeated; then the opposite can happen: the information gets stronger. This concept has been around for more than 200 years and has been tested in clinical practice by thousands of doctors. The idea was first launched by Dr Samuel Hahnemann, who invented homeopathy, the first Western science to apply the principles of quantum physics long before they were discovered and researched.

MIASMAS: ENERGETIC IMPURITIES

Dr Samuel Hahnemann called the cell-memory he discovered *miasma*. 'Miasma' means impurity; 'miasmal' means pathogenic (disease-causing). We could use this term for all the pathogenic information that people inherit from previous generations, and this also accounts for the miasmal information collected during a lifetime that remains detectable long after the origin of the disease or symptoms have disappeared. This information is stored in an electromagnetic resonance manner. It can be latent until activated or brought to the fore by certain incidents creating an electromagnetic signal on the same wavelength and influencing cellular processes, leading to changes in specific organs or tissues. This is very similar to the way dormant viruses are activated. The difference is that a real virus has its information coded in the DNA or RNA, while miasmic information does not have a representation in matter, it is just information logged into the system. Miasma correlates, to a certain extent, to what could be called family-karma or blood-karma. This is the karma we apparently choose or assume by incarnating into a specific family. We will have their genetic and constitutional strengths (positive karma), but also their genetic and constitutional weaknesses (negative karma).

Miasma is always *negative karma* – but the good news is that it can always be eradicated through emotional balance and homeopathy. Some forms of meditation and Qigong can help as well.

REPROGRAMMABLE DNA: THE SCIENCE OF EPIGENETICA

Let's look further into cell-memory. The original cell-memory (programming) is in the DNA (deoxyribonucleic acid) and in its mirror twin, RNA (ribonucleic acid). DNA is where spirit and matter meet. Spirit expresses itself through our DNA. DNA without spirit is just a strand of nucleic acids; chemicals with no power whatsoever. Through the blessing of spirit, the DNA becomes the most advanced team of engineers that can build anything from scratch, using the simplest building blocks – mainly amino acids and water. They have in store all the blueprints of all the organs and tissues in your body. It has your personality type, your basic patterns of thinking, already programmed. By accessing your consciousness, you can change these programs and influence your DNA.

There is a dynamic exchange between anti-matter (spirit) and matter, and this exchange occurs through your DNA. Nothing happens in your body without the involvement of your DNA. It is the servant of your divine intelligence, your connection to the Source of it all. All the matter that represents you, with all your senses and brain capacity, has been created through your DNA. A great deal of our programming for health, disease and longevity is based in our DNA. The good news is that we can influence DNA to work for us. By visualizing a positive, happy, healthy and vital future we will activate the chromosomes on the corresponding DNA, and block the DNA parts that promote disease, degeneration and premature ageing. The trick is to focus only on the end result. In this way you will erase or overwrite what your subconscious mind has already gathered throughout the years. This is called *epigenetica*.

Emotional DNA

Richard Turner introduced the term 'emotional DNA' in one of his publications. It is about emotional programming and cell-memory. Some interesting work in emotional memory is done through hypnosis. In a procedure called regression hypnosis, a person is first brought under hypnosis, then is asked to go back in time. People have been known to re-experience accurately any period of their lives, with details that they cannot consciously remember under normal circumstances. They can tell you exactly what clothes they wore on their third birthday, the presents they received, all the people who were there and more. Somehow the mind registers everything we experience and stores it. Asking where someone was before being in this body provides some interesting stories. It is similar to near-death experiences, in which people are clinically dead or going through severe trauma during which they experience a glimpse of the 'other side'. All subjects tell similar stories of another realm totally different from our reality. In this realm other entities exist as well and some sort of coaching, evaluation and teaching.

Reincarnation or Dream Time?

When asked to go back further in time, most people will encounter other lives they have lived. They can convey details of this former life as if living it right now, and sometimes speak foreign languages fluently. Does this prove reincarnation? Maybe it does, maybe it doesn't. If you do not want to believe, that's OK as there is no tangible evidence. Reincarnation as a general philosophy is neither Christian nor anti-Christian. It is not a religion but just a philosophical idea that can help us understand our lives better. It can be incorporated into many different religions without taking anything away from them. Just as chakras and meridians are concepts that can help you access more of your potential, you can be open to the theory of reincarnation and still practise Christianity, Judaism, Hinduism or Buddhism. In my clinical practice I try to stay away from the idea of reincarnation if the patient's beliefs do not allow it, and that is fine. But if a patient is open to believing, I can access information from previous lives, if needed, to find out the cause of a current problem. What is interesting is that all of this information is saved in our cell-memory; details of hundreds of lives, some short, some very short and some longer.

An alternative theory is that we dream in metaphors, so it could be that we dream as if we have lived before and this is stored in our memory banks as reality. You can believe that if it feels better. I am sure we can come up with other theories as well; I am not interested in proving or disproving any of them – I am interested in getting results and helping people heal and have happy, healthy lives.

Personally I have come to believe in reincarnation as part of the infinite, ongoing cycle of our immortal souls. With each passing from physical life, when we let go of the conscious mind which is connected with our material existence, we have the opportunity to evaluate our progress and access our needs for further spiritual growth. Every time we leave our physical body, we enter a heightened state of awareness and come closer to our core soul-identity so we can experience our true purpose. The Earth holds the lessons that we can learn in a three- (sometimes four-) dimensional material classroom. There are also other planes of consciousness where we undergo other kinds of development and learning. One reason for coming back is to pick up where we left off in our last life. For that reason much of our turbulence in this life is the result of unfinished business in previous lives. The good news is that it does not matter whether you believe in previous lives or not; the soul's purpose remains the same.

WE ALL HAVE ONE PURPOSE IN COMMON

That purpose is to let go of old patterns which make us turn away from our ultimate goal: *the state of unconditional love and living in the moment without bias or judgement.* Each moment we experience gives us the chance to be in the present and to make choices based on our highest values and not on the past. As soon as we let go of that pattern, we no longer attract that situation or it no longer saps our energy. Universal love is mirrored in the law of cause and effect to guide us to a deeper understanding on the soul level of our experiences in materiality. The most beautiful aspect of this which has become clear for me, working with thousands of patients, is that the story of the soul on our plane of existence is the story of a loving God who never ceases to give His/Her children the chance to wake up to who they really are. That is the only reason why we experience inner turmoil or turbulence.

Each time we experience stress, pain or discomfort, it's a wake-up call to look inside.

The theory of reincarnation does not answer all questions; it mainly addresses the law of karma and the possibility of spiritual development through the cycle of rebirth. The deeper we go into understanding this, the more questions will arise that cannot be answered.

Here are some questions that may intrigue you:

- *When does the soul enter the body?*

From testing patients I've learned that, from the moment of conception, the spirit claims the body and stays connected with it. The physical body can pick up all kinds of experiences that do not come from the soul. Most of these experiences and memories are tied into those of the mother. This needs to be cleansed later from the cell-memory. Normally this happens naturally, but when the child grows up and its basic needs are not met, many of these memories will persist and we may carry with us emotions picked up from our mother. In the majority of cases, the soul's entry occurs at some point before birth or at birth.

- ● **How often does the soul come back to Earth?**

There is no average for anyone; there are great variations. There is no set interval between lives; sometimes a person may come back just shortly after dying or may stay without incarnating for thousands of years.

CORE CELL-MEMORY

There are many more questions my patients ask me about this; let's put some things into place that relate to cell-memory and its consequences in our lives by taking a look at where the information comes from that is part of our core cell-memory:

- ● while in the womb, starting at conception
- ● in the 'astral' period before incarnation (in between lives)
- ● from miasmas, inherited information of previous generations
- ● from previous lives
- ● information picked up during sleep
- ● information from daydreams or visualizations
- ● via telepathy and other ways we pick up information from the morphogenetic field or from others we are in contact with
- ● information we pick up from other people directly
- ● information we get from organ transplants

Let's look at these one by one and see how they can affect our emotional balance.

In the Womb

The developing foetus is like a crystal or a CD-rom. Quantum physics has proven that water and crystals function like memory chips. The developing foetus is the same. Things said by the mother or people directly in her environment can be picked up and stored. This is called 'prenatal text'. This term has been coined by psychotherapist Loek Knippels, a friend of mine. Years later someone can be triggered emotionally by hearing the same words or sentences. Also, this text can come back to haunt you as part of your own inner dialogue. This is similar to the experiences people have when they undergo surgery under anaesthesia. There is a part of their minds always actively listening to what the surgeons and nurses are saying. Negative remarks during surgery can cause deep emotional wounds or traumas that may affect the person's recovery and future for good. The same thing happens during pregnancy: even though the baby or foetus may not be neurologically mature enough to understand meaning, the intention and the sentences are stored. Scientific research has shown that talking to a developing foetus in the womb and playing classical or new age music has a positive effect on the delivery and also on the immune system and adaptability of the newborn. This can only be explained if we let go of the idea that the central nervous system is the only place where we store information.

CASE STUDY: PRENATAL MEMORY

Jill was a typical 16-year-old: every imaginable body part pierced, including her tongue, ears, navel, nipples and eyebrows. The reason her mother brought her to see me was Jill's self-destructive behaviour. She smoked, drank, drove recklessly and was a daredevil of whom even her 17-year-old brother was frightened. She had broken many bones, including her nose, elbows, ankles, four vertebrae, ribs, etc. She seemed to take pleasure in coming home with something broken or out of place. It was a miracle she was still alive. The family had tried three psychologists and three psychiatrists, to no avail. By the magic of coincidence I had been seated next to her father on a transatlantic flight. When he'd seen me writing for hours during the flight, he'd asked me what I was doing. 'I am writing a book,' I'd replied. 'About what?' he'd asked. I'd told him I was writing a book on phobias and other emotional problems and how to cure them rapidly instead of with complicated psychotherapy. After a while he'd spoken about his serious concerns regarding his teenage daughter. I'd told him I do not take on new patients because of my busy schedule, but that I was willing to look into it and offer some advice.

Jill was the third child, her brother was one year older and her oldest sister was 23 years old, married and, like her brother, well behaved. Her father was a well-to-do developer with projects all over Florida. They were constantly embarrassed by their daughter's behaviour. I did my usual tests on her to find out, first, if there were any factors that could explain her erratic behaviour such as low blood sugar, allergies, chemical toxins, electro-smog or chronic infections; all of these tested negative. Then I started an emotional screening using predominantly muscle-testing and questions. Within five minutes I had located her emotional trauma.

Three weeks after conception, Jill's mother had discovered, to her dismay, that she was pregnant. She was not happy at all as it was not planned and she had actually wanted only two children. She considered and discussed abortion as an option with her husband, but accepted the pregnancy because of her religious beliefs. Jill had locked in on the fact that she was unwanted and that her parents had thought about killing her. So, in her own way, she was still trying to abort herself because she felt that she did not deserve to live. Her mother started to cry when I revealed what I'd found, and in her own words repeated the whole story. She asked her daughter for forgiveness. After that I balanced the disturbed meridians and the first chakra. After this treatment, Jill changed completely, not only in her behaviour but also in her looks, her dress-code and friends. This is the power of 'prenatal text'.

The 'Astral Period' Before Incarnation

It is not my intention to prove to anyone that we reincarnate or that we are immortal souls. I am a clinician and a researcher; I get tough cases to solve and that forces me to look for answers where most doctors don't tread. I only have one goal in mind and that is to support my patients' healing in the most natural way possible. I have been very successful and have taught the insights of my research to doctors, health professionals and laypeople worldwide. The 'astral period' is a cell-memory that all of us carry inside ourselves. During this period we decide the purpose of our coming to this material plane and what we want to learn to get closer to the highest and purest vibration of love possible. Findings in thousands of patients have led me to believe that the purpose of our being here is *to discover our real potential by letting go of all the unnecessary pain and suffering that we create by not understanding who we really are*. We don't have to learn anything; we just have to realize that love is the answer, no matter what the question.

CASE STUDY: ASTRAL MEMORY

Ann was 37 years old and came to me for depression and suicidal thoughts. She had been seeing a psychiatrist who had put her on Prozac. She felt better but her real problem was that she kept being with men who abused her. In these destructive relationships she would repeatedly sacrifice her own needs for her lover's selfish demands. When I asked her if she believed in reincarnation, she was not sure. She'd never really given it any thought. The reason she had become particularly depressed was that she'd found herself attracted to a very abusive man. For some strange reason she kept going back to him. We decided to explore a possible past-life connection with muscle-testing. In this way we discovered that the man had been her father in a previous life and had been abusive at that time as well. She could now understand that the anger from her father in that life came from the fact that her mother had died giving birth to her. Her father blamed her and physically abused her any chance he could get. During her 'astral period', she and this man connected to come back and find a way to forgive each other.

At the end of the testing we did a forgiveness-session, in which she forgave herself for having caused the death of another person and for the grief her previous father had endured because of that. She also forgave her lover for abusing her. She cried tears of relief and left feeling light and optimistic. She called me up the next week to tell me that something strange happened: when she'd got home, she'd found her lover crying and asking her for forgiveness. He had been home watching a talk show while she was with me. On the talk show the subject was 'Why women love men who abuse them'. Their relationship changed instantly and she no longer needed anti-depressants. When she hung up I stared silently into space, completely puzzled by the workings of the universe. I had known for a long time that there are no coincidences, but every time synchronicity takes its course, I'm amazed by the grace of our collective consciousness. We have all this information accessible to us in our core cell-memory, and it is not difficult to access it.

Miasmas

Miasma is pathogenic inherited information that can affect our health and emotional balance. Miasmas can be imprinted by a wide variety of causes, such as suppressed infections, toxins such as chemicals or heavy metals, vaccinations and unresolved emotions. All of these are becoming more and more common in our modern times due to the exaggerated use of antibiotics, immunizations and the increasingly ubiquitous pollution. In chronic disease we often find miasmas as one of the most crippling factors for the immune system. The most encountered miasmas are emotional. By eliminating the miasmas, we create more 'breathing space' for the immune system, so it can do its job better. Miasmas can affect our emotional state as well, as the following case study demonstrates.

CASE STUDY: MIASMAL MEMORY

Rick was a 19-year-old boy who consulted me for severe allergies which had resulted in bronchitis and sinusitis. He was now studying medicine and his father was a cardiologist. His father did not approve of him visiting me, but his mother,

Millie, knew me very well and brought him anyway. When he was a child, Rick had had asthmatic bronchitis and would get panic attacks. He would scream and shout in terror and repeatedly say, 'I am going to die!' He saw the best doctors in the country and got a lot of medication, including corticosteroids. The family had got rid of all pets and carpets, and relocated twice to areas that would be better for him. Around the age of eight, the attacks became less and less frequent, then totally disappeared at age 11. He became hyperactive at the age of nine and addicted to all sorts of junk food.

I started my work-up on him and quickly found that his allergies were emotional and the main governing emotion was grief. I traced it back to a miasma from his mother's side. I tracked it three generations back. His mother's grandmother had suffered some great loss connected with losing a child just after birth. Millie was perplexed at my diagnosis but she recalled that her mother has suffered from postnatal depression, as had she. She also knew the story about her grandmother to be correct. When Rick was born, she was in a deep postnatal depression and what got her out of it was when Rick got severe bronchitis when he was two months old and was hospitalized. Rick subconsciously developed the notion that he would only get attention if he was ill. He felt rejected by his mother because she did not really take care of him as a baby. A nanny took care of him and he was not breastfed. Probably because of the effect on his immune system, he quickly developed allergies to milk and, later, to other foods.

I worked with Rick to assist him in letting go of all the grief and hurt he carried with him. Millie also got three sessions to let go of her own grief. Two months later she brought her mother, who had just turned 70, in for a visit. She had taken anti-depressants for more than 15 years. I treated her for six sessions before she was ready to let go of her inheritance. This exceptional family session could have ended here but, to my surprise, Rick's father, the cardiologist, came to see me one day to thank me for all I had done for his family. Rick had been symptom-free for over a year and Millie was singing in the shower, something she had never before done in her whole life.

Previous Existences

The philosophy of reincarnation is being embraced by more and more people in Western society. Celebrities and other well-known public figures speak openly about it, it is discussed on television talk shows and features as the subject of many movies and books, including some bestsellers. We can now talk about it even with people who for religious reasons are not allowed to consider it a possibility. There are many past-life workshops and regression hypnotherapies. The good thing about the idea of reincarnation is that it encourages people to take responsibility for their development as spiritual beings with a specific mission to accomplish. It can offer us meaning where it is difficult to see any sense. When children suffer or people die in seemingly senseless accidents, this philosophy may offer hope or insight. Most of us assume that death of the physical body is bad. When we look at the information we get from people who have had a so-called near-death experience, regression hypnosis or clairvoyant episodes, the message is always the same: life without a physical body is interestingly enjoyable. The question is, if somehow we do have control of our reality and from a higher, conscious state we make the decision to leave this life, is that wrong? There are a variety of reasons to leave and many to stay as well. No one can make that decision for anyone else. The common things that people say such as 'He was still so young' or 'He had everything going for him' or 'She was in the prime of her life' are no match for other deeply personal objectives known only to the Higher Self of the person involved and which relate to the much larger issue of the purpose of his or her life in terms of consciousness, karma and growth.

There are times when we are faced with an extreme and very dramatic event. Often there have been signals we've ignored along the way. Any traumatic incident offers many advanced lessons to all involved. It forces us to look at our path and make new choices. In the end, as I've said before, it does not really matter if you believe in reincarnation or not. What is there will be there. In my work this concept makes sense and has helped thousands of people. I want to share a personal story with you that made me open my eyes to these other possibilities.

MY STORY

As a child, I too suffered from asthmatic bronchitis. Every time I suffered an attack, I had the sensation of dying and being asphyxiated. At times I would gasp for air like a fish on land, and turn blue. I had an intense fear of being alone and during an attack I would panic totally. The medical doctors could only offer some relief but not a total cure. My grandmother, who knew something about herbs, treated me and gradually, after four years of suffering, the attacks abated. I was around seven at the time. After that I became hyperactive and suffered from Attention Deficit Disorder (ADD). In spite of this I was very committed to learning and, miraculously, made it through schools with exceptional grades. In the meantime I suffered from hypoglycaemia, allergies, eczema, sinusitis, insomnia, migraines, recurrent viral infections, chronic fatigue, muscle cramps, dizziness and fainting. I made it through medical school thanks to my dedication to the martial arts. One year after graduating as an MD, I embarked on researching and studying alternative medicine to find my own cure. A strange phenomenon was that I had an aversion to the German language and to Germans. Living in the Netherlands during my medical studies, I'd had to go to Germany on several occasions for martial arts competitions. I always felt uncomfortable and would come back with headaches. The reason for this became clear to me only after I underwent a session of regression hypnosis.

During this session I recalled being a Jewish boy of 16 who was taken to a concentration camp in Germany and who had perished there with thousand others in the gas chambers. I experienced my death, which was very frightening, and my transcendence to another realm. After this session many things changed in my life; most of my allergies were gone, and my aversion to Germans and the German language was gone, too. Whether it was true or not, many things and feelings in my life made much more sense, and ever since I have been dedicated to finding a way that can be used by everyone to let go of issues from their past, no matter if they came about in previous lives or this one. I think I have succeeded, as you will learn in Part II of this book.

In many cultures, reincarnation is an accepted philosophy and is ingrained in people's lives. In India there have been many documented cases of children who can remember exactly what happened to them in previous lives. Some murder cases have been solved after children have been able to point out who killed them in a previous life. Scientists do not believe that these cases prove reincarnation. So let's reveal other possibilities for these déjà vu experiences:

- The subconscious picks up information from the morphogenetic field and experiences this as its own reality.
- The subconscious identifies with a certain person from the past. Many people under hypnosis will say they were, for example, Napoleon or Joan of Arc in a previous life.
- The subconscious translates incidents and occurrences in daily life symbolically (in metaphor) and accepts these metaphors as the truth.
- During our sleep we experience other lives in our dreams or through out-of-body experiences and these are recorded by the brain as real events.
- People pick up on events that have happened to other people and store these as if they'd happened to them.

There must be other possibilities as well, and also combinations of the above, including reincarnation. It is also possible that time is not linear as we experience it, but that different things happen simultaneously and that our souls can connect with these parallel realities. To be honest, it is not even important to know about all this; it does not make any difference to the outcome. The only time I discuss it in clinical practice is when it can give someone added insights that can speed up their recovery, or when a patient has questions that I cannot answer in any other way.

Information Picked Up During Sleep

During our sleep we are not idle. There is the possibility that our soul is somewhere else. This 'somewhere else' is not necessary in our material 3-D dimension. Some of these adventures are to be found in dreams, some do not leave any conscious recollection. Prof. Tiller in his book *The Science of Human Transformation* discusses scientific reasons to assume there is a dimension parallel to ours, which he refers to as anti-matter or ether. In this dimension information travels faster than light. This relates to the *Siddhi* state of consciousness.

CASE STUDY

I have a very good friend who is a Belgian homeopath by the name of Carina. I visited her about 16 years ago and met her daughter Chiara, who was three years old at the time. We had an instant rapport and, strangely, for the next three years Chiara would appear regularly in my dreams saying, 'Roy, let's play!' and off we would go playing in the fields. Another strange thing was that Carina told me that Chiara, after meeting me, spoke about me every day. One time I was talking to Carina while preparing notes for a book called *Vitality Medicine*; I was doing some research on these phenomena. I asked Carina to ask Chiara what she was doing every night when she went to sleep. The answer was: 'Every night I go to play with Roy!' I am sure there may be other explanations for this, but I have this very strong feeling that at least a part of my dreamtime I spend with Chiara. In my clinical practice I do not make use of this knowledge at this time. I keep it as a possibility in the back of my head, and if it proves useful in some case I will certainly look into it.

Information from Daydreams or Visualizations

Every thought that is charged with enough emotion will be recorded as part of our emotional reality. If you spend time thinking about something for long enough, it will become part of you. The same goes for visualizations: the more vivid and multi-sensorial they are, the greater the chance that they will become reality.

There is a story that I love to tell because it has impressed me so much and actually was the reason I really got into this direction. I had used visualizations unknowingly for quite some time in martial arts. Before each championship I would picture myself winning and receiving the honours related to that. I remained undefeated European champion for 150 consecutive bouts. In 1989 I really got interested in visualizations because of what my then-partner Erica told me. She said that if you visualize with all your senses (smell, taste, sight, hearing and touch), you will manifest what you want much faster. I decided to visualize something that would be impossible. I visualized that someone would give me a car. Not just any car, an expensive sportscar. I had a picture of the make and model I wanted, one I was sure I would never be able to buy. For 10 minutes every day I would imagine sitting in the car, smelling the leather, feeling the steering wheel and driving the car. I did this for four months (yes, I wanted that car!). Nothing happened. Around the summer of 1989 I took an assignment to help build the most advanced clinic for alternative medicine in Switzerland. When we arrived there to live for a few years to supervise the project, something strange happened. The person in charge of the project came to me and said, 'Dr Martina, you'll need a car and one of my managers just quit and we still have a year's lease on the car, why don't you take it?' He walked me over to the car and I was totally flabbergasted: not only was it the make of car I'd visualized, it was the same model, even the same colour. The first thought that crossed my mind was, *You fool, why didn't you visualize an even more expensive one?!*

I am a true believer in visualization and I normally achieve all the things I visualize – some of them with some delay but I know that in due time, if I engrain it in my subconscious mind, it will come to me!

Telepathy

Psychic phenomena such as telepathy and clairvoyance occur more frequently than we know. We've learned to ignore the signs and not to accept their validity. The subconscious sometimes cannot tell the difference between its own memory and what it is picking up from elsewhere.

CASE STUDY: TELEPATHY

Mrs Lindsay came to see me because she was having abdominal pains on her right side, in the region of her gallbladder. Several tests by her internist could not find anything and she'd received all sorts of medication that did not help. She was 56 years old and had been suffering for three months. I started to test her and found that the pain she was experiencing was, according to my findings, emotional. But the peculiar thing was that she had picked this up from her daughter. Her daughter was suffering from a physical gallbladder problem that was caused by her frustration with her marriage. Mrs Lindsay was completely shocked by my diagnosis; she told me that everything I'd told her was correct and that her daughter was going to have surgery the following week for gallstones. She had never linked the two things together. The peculiar thing was that her daughter had started to feel ill only two weeks previously!

I gave Mrs Lindsay an acupuncture treatment and some flower remedies. Her pains went away after the treatment. This is not an exceptional case; it happens more often than you think. Her daughter lived far away from her and they spoke on the phone once a week.

I have seen similar cases where people pick up information even from objects such as jewellery, watches and rings. The strangest one was a woman suffering from severe headaches and migraines resulting from the energy she was picking up from a portrait of her grandfather hanging in her living room. After my consultation she called up her mother, who confirmed that her grandfather had suffered from headaches. This woman had been using painkillers for 12 years. I have seen cases where imbalances result from wearing jewellery that once belonged to someone else. Certain people can pick up information about the people they are in contact with and pass it on to others.

As you can see, we have to become aware of what is happening in ourselves; we cannot take anything for granted. You can even pick up information from places, especially if there has been some sort of traumatic emotional event there, such as a death or murder.

Information from Others

This is much more common and we have all experienced it. Sometimes you talk to someone who is in deep pain, is grieving or depressed, etc. After the conversation you take away with you a depressed feeling you cannot shake. In some cases this can last for days. Normally it happens with people with whom we sympathize. The bad news is that we can pick things up from complete strangers. What you need to know about this sort of reactions is that it can only happen if you have some similar unresolved issues in your system. Then you resonate with their disharmonious vibrations. By working on your issues, this will happen less and less often.

CASE STUDY: PICKING UP EMOTIONS

When my oldest son Sunray was four, he became very hyperactive. At that time he was under the care of a babysitter for two nights a week. He did not want to sleep and would not listen to any of the things that his mother Erica or I told him. I tested him and found that he picked up frustration from the babysitter. This energy completely disrupted his balance and caused the hyperactive behaviour. After treating the gallbladder and liver acupoints, he returned to the normal behaviour to which we were accustomed. The babysitter always had headphones on and her music was loud; I remembered that I'd asked her not to wear headphones when she babysat and she'd given me one of those irritated looks that made me decide not to ask her again. After treating Sunray, everything fell into place.

Many doctors and therapists are very tired after seeing patients all day. I know this feeling very well. What I discovered is that we resonate so much with many of our patients' emotional pathology that it drains our life-force. By being aware of this and treating ourselves with the protocols in this book, the problem disappears completely and at the end of the day we can feel refreshed and energized. This is important for anyone who works with people or is in contact with different people during the course of a day.

Information from Organ Transplants

When an organ is transplanted, more is passed on than just the physical organ. The cell-memory of the donor is passed on as well. I have no personal experience of patients who have been recipients of another's organs or tissues, but what I have seen in the literature and heard from fellow doctors is that in several cases the recipient experiences changes in behaviour and even develops cravings. In Dr Paul Pearsall's bestselling book *The Heart's Code*, a story is described of a woman who received a heart transplant. Shortly afterwards she dreamed about a young man who mentioned his name and thanked her for taking care of his heart. She then experienced cravings for hamburgers and beer, something she never had before her surgery. She went to the library to research the obituaries of the dates just before her transplant and found the name of the person who'd appeared in her dream. She tracked the family down and found out that he had liked hamburgers and beer. This is evidence that more is going on than meets the eye.

After reading this chapter I hope you have an idea of the possible perturbations of our emotional balance we can sometimes face. Despite the overwhelming possibilities around cell-memory, the overall good news is that in most instances we can take control and solve the underlying causes of our emotional turbulence.

Part II

Emotional Balance

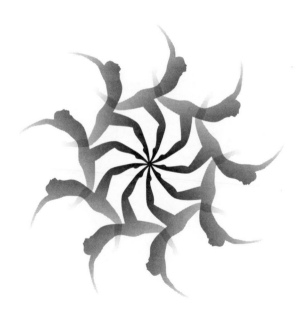

CHAPTER 8

THE 14 GATEWAYS TO EMOTIONAL BALANCE

EMOTIONAL BALANCE POINTS AND TOTAL HEALTH

We have the tendency to regard the mind and body as two separate entities; this in itself creates a blockage of energy flow in the meridians. We may say things like, 'My back is killing me,' 'I can't stand this pain in my shoulder' or 'My head is hurting.' By formulating our ailments in this way we are isolating those affected parts from our emotional energy. By isolating affected parts we create the opposite of what we want. The physical body is an expression of our internal world. Every little or big symptom has a deeper underlying reason. A spot, a rash, a pain, itching, etc. are all signs that we need to look within. Instead of seeking a quick panacea, we should engage in the art of communication with ourselves.

A friend of mine, Jan van den Burg, gives an example of this. He is a marketing expert from the Netherlands and was giving a presentation to the board of a big corporation in Paris. The second day of the meeting he woke up with a high fever, sore throat and hoarse voice. Jan has been to many of my seminars and workshops, and has always been very creative with the material. He lay down and began to relax and meditate. Then he entered into communication with his subconscious mind. He said, 'I know you have a perfect reason for doing what you are doing now, and I thank you for taking such good care of my body and me. I want to ask you a big favour: could you put what you're doing on hold or slow it down, so I can finish my presentation? I only need three more hours!' He meditated for another half-hour, and by the time he came out of meditation his fever was gone, his voice was clear and he felt OK. Not terrific, but good enough to do what he had to do. He returned to his room three hours later after a great presentation and a contract. He went to bed and immediately his fever came back. He treated the EB (emotional balance) points and the next day he was back to normal. This is, in principle, what we all need to learn: to deal with our body in a respectful way that will honour us. That is the real magic we must learn if we are to take physical and emotional responsibility for our own wellbeing. We live in a culture where millions do not deal with their own issues. They use chemicals, drugs, herbs, vitamins, medical doctors and alternative health practitioners to create more and more suppression of their body's healing capacities. To go to Level 3 of creation – the magical, effortless approach – we need to discover and experience the total intertwined spiral of physical body, feelings, emotions, spirit and mind. All of this, all the time, for all of who we are. To find emotional balance, the state of flow, we must combine the yang (head) and the yin (heart) to get to *Tao*. Tao (pronounced 'dow') in Chinese literally means 'the Way', the effortless path followed by all of the universe, the structure in the chaos, the underlying intelligence that many refer to as God. Tao is the ultimate reality, the essence of Nature. It is the gateway to all that is, all that can be seen and cannot be seen. Lao Tzu writes in the opening words of the *Tao Te Ching*: 'The Tao that can be experienced is not the eternal Tao. The Tao is absolute and infinite, whereas words are relative and limited. Words are mere boxes which cannot contain entire visions of Tao, but only parts of that vision.' This was written in 500 BC; the name Lao Tzu means 'old man', indicating that the author(s) is unknown.

The basic principles of emotional balance come from many philosophies and sciences, but in the end only one goal remains and that is to find the harmony in your reality. In Part I we read about unresolved emotions, triggers, self-rejection and emotional blocks to healing, karma, chakras and cell-memory to understand what we are facing. Here in Part II we will look at the tools and techniques we will utilize to create emotional balance.

Emotional balance gives us the opportunity to get out of the vortex of our emotional turmoil and find our still-point, the zone of harmonious flow. We live in an unseen, unheard universe of electromagnetic fields, and we are ourselves radiant examples of energy vibration. Every unresolved emotion creates a disharmonious pattern of energy that we radiate out into the universe. By this mechanism we attract and repel other people with similar or opposite energy patterns. If you have a problem with trusting people, you will attract people who will prove to you that you are right: you cannot trust anyone. Balancing our disharmonious energies creates a shift in our energy fields and we will attract other people who will fit our energies better. We've already read about how unresolved emotions turn against us and destroy our physical body. We have also seen that our self-image, the concept we have about ourselves, will determine our success. We have learned that the chakras play a key role in our emotional patterns and behaviour. And, most importantly, we have realized how much rubbish we take with us from previous generations, previous lives and more.

WHAT DO WE NEED TO ACHIEVE EMOTIONAL BALANCE?

How do we let go of our emotional baggage? Our response to any given situation is based mainly on the past; we need to change this and respond in the present moment.

The 14 gateways to balance are special acupoints that were discovered over 5,000 years ago.

Knowing these 14 points is like having access to the mainframe computer. It is the key to changing the programming of our emotions and behaviour.

What makes emotional balancing different from other forms of psychotherapy is that it focuses only on the feelings. By focusing on our feelings, we open up to the intentions of our spirit. What gets in our way is past unresolved issues, which literally shut down the flow of energy. By focusing on what we are feeling, we can evaluate the reason why we are feeling it and react accordingly.

Let's take the following example: you are in conversation with a friend and talking about intimate issues of life. All of a sudden you feel some discomfort in your neck area. Still carrying on with the conversation, you massage your neck with one hand, without giving any thought to the why this is happening. After the conversation you feel drained and you have a headache. There is tension in your body; if you are like a million other people, you will take something for your headache and get on with your life. You will have missed a chance to tune in to the magnificent apparatus that your body is. If you keep doing this, sooner or later your body will malfunction and you will have become hostage to all the unresolved issues stored in your cell-memory.

What's the solution? By using 14 special points on the body, we can balance all of the tensions we experience. We can go to any given situation in the past and clear up any lingering emotional residue of the past. For emotional balancing it does not matter if a trauma is severe or not; if a phobia is very intense or if we believe what is done to us is insurmountable or unforgivable. On an energetic level all of these distinctions and qualifications totally disappear, and the question is simple: does the energy flow unhindered or not? If it is hindered, there is a blockage. It really does not matter if the blockage is large or small; the principles for treating a life-disturbing phobia about leaving the house or just a little bit of anxiety about leaving the house are exactly the same. The only difference is in someone's mind. The type of labels we put on our experiences will become our reality.

Let's take an example: two people have to give a speech for the first time to quite a large audience. Both of them feel sensations in their stomach area and tension in the area of the neck, eyes and throat. The only difference will be what they are thinking. One thinks that he may forget everything, look ridiculous, lose face and make a fool of himself. He will start feeling worse and worse, and eventually may create that reality. But even in the event that none of that happens and the speech goes fine, next time he will experience very similar sensations. I once met a psychologist who, like me, was a guest speaker at a medical convention. She was terrified and had to take calming pills before she could go on stage. Once on stage she was totally paralyzed and she read from her notes for 30 minutes without once making eye-contact with the audience. After my lecture she came to me and said, 'I envy you; you are so calm and confident, how do you do it?' She was 64 years old and highly respected for her many books and research. She had been given lectures for over 20 years, on average twice a month. Each time she would be terrified and unable to sleep for two nights before giving the lecture. After a 10-minute session with emotional balancing, her fear of public speaking disappeared forever. Going back to our example, suppose the other speaker feels the same sensations but labels them completely differently. He says to himself, 'I feel these sensations because I am excited, I am ready, I feel that this will be a great lecture – I can't wait to get on stage!' His experience will be totally different. So, the way we label our sensations will create the reality that we experience. The key is to get to the raw, unfiltered sensation and work from there. Working with the meridians enables us to let go of the past and burn karma through resolving issues that have kept us trapped in karmic patterns. *Emotional Balancing is one of the fastest ways to burn karma and stay in the present.*

YIN – YANG – TAO

Harmony is the result of synergy between the two fundamental principles of energy and emotions. Emotions, whether expressed or not, should be integrated and released. Emotions are the charge our mind gives to feeling. This charge is the result of our subconscious mind, which relates the situation or feeling to perceived danger. *Integration means acceptance of the feeling without the charge.*

In other words, we accept and acknowledge that we feel a certain way, and consciously we receive the message of our subconscious mind. It is like saying, 'Thank you for warning me, I have seen the danger and I will stay alert!'

Once we've acknowledged the message, there is no need to hold on to it and we can let it go. Letting go means taking responsibility and being ready for action based on the incoming information. We stay relaxed and ready. This technique of *integration* and *release* is the basis of many Eastern health systems and martial arts. In martial arts, I teach my students to become one with their opponent, integrating their energy field with their opponent's and releasing all fears. By synchronizing ourselves with the perceived enemy, we no longer have an enemy and we are dealing only with energy, nothing else. We can feel the energy and change its direction so it will not harm us. If we do not synchronize we will be tense and use more energy, and as such fall victim to our fears.

- Yang = the charge we give to a sensation, based on the present
- Yin = the meaning we give to the sensation based on the past
- Tao = synergy, returning to the flow state or natural state of being, one with all there is.

CHI-FLOW

Our goal is awareness and being in the present. Emotional balancing will teach us how to become more aware of tensions, blocks and inhibitions, and also to integrate these and let go of them. This will bring us to a whole new level of experiencing the Chi-flow through our bodies and thus get in touch with our inner self, which allows us to connect with every cell in our body. Our concept of who we are will gradually change as our energy body expands, our mind expands and we start feeling more of a unity between mind, body and spirit. We will gradually learn to find the path of intuition and least resistance and start manifesting our *Siddhi* consciousness. This is where we feel the energetic connections that exist between ourselves and all beings in Nature, and eventually with all beings in the universe. We feel the universal energy which no longer separates the 'I' from the rest. Now we can utilize what has been there but has never been made manifest. You will raise your energy levels to unknown heights because no longer will you let your life-force ebb or be sapped by others, or used to push against resistance from your past. Your energy abundance will lead to health and vitality and will illuminate any place you are and support the healing of others. You will no longer be infected with the emotional viruses of others, such as anxiety, paranoia, fears, worries, low self-esteem, grief, depression and suspicion, but you will stay connected with your inner self.

EMOTIONAL BALANCE AND VULNERABILITY

There is much confusion about vulnerability, which is seen by many as an unwanted quality. The opposite of vulnerability is creating emotional armour, which always results in chronic physical tension. The body will lock painful memories in certain areas and link them to certain parts of our physiology. This will foster, or in some cases trigger, certain emotions that had nothing to do with the original incident or event. This can also lead to changes in the body such as habitually hunching the shoulders, stiffness in the joints or tension in the muscles. Resisting feelings makes the emotion persistent. *What you resist persists.* You end up feeding the unwanted sensations with energy, which only makes them stronger.

By the time we become aware of what we are feeling it is already causing tension, energy blocks, soreness and so on. The essence of 'emotional armour' is an attempt to anaesthetize ourselves to unpleasant feelings; in reality, though, we become their slaves. Being vulnerable means accepting the feelings, becoming comfortable with feeling uncomfortable or *feeling good about feeling bad.* Emotions and feelings can enrich our lives, when we stay balanced.

EMOTIONAL ARMOUR IS COUNTERPRODUCTIVE

The more we try to suppress what we feel, the more blockages we create, the more turbulence we experience in the form of depression, irritation, anxiety, discontentment and frustration. These unwanted feelings creep into your day, your mornings, your relationships, your marriage, your work, your evenings and even your sleep. You wake up feeling most unlike a million dollars and with a sensation of impending doom. You lose sight of all the things you have going for you; you don't see the little things anymore and gradually lose life-force and zest for life. You may seek out cigarettes, sugar- or salt-laden snacks, television, trashy magazines, talking too much, drinking too much or taking drugs or medication in order to try to calm down again. You cease to grow and get stuck in survival mode. This is karmic waste.

Vulnerability seems scary to many people, but it really is about self-awareness and will lead to freedom. Self-awareness is being in touch with your spirit, which is your connection to universal energy. By acknowledging the feelings we can become more alert to our spiritual path and constantly move toward still-point. Still-point is where there is inner peace. When we make choices and evaluations from still-point, we are choosing without the unresolved karma from the past. We are connected with the spirit and not the ego. In this way we can choose based on our uninhibited intuition and find the path that will not create new karmic debt. This path is *dharma* (Sanskrit) or *chosaku* (Japanese): the path of magic, the path of bliss and effortlessness. Effortlessness does not mean that we do nothing; it means we do not lose life-force or create new unwanted luggage (negative karma). It means letting go of all that weighs you down, that creates inner turmoil or turbulence.

Vulnerability is the state of openness, the state of connecting to the self: knowing who you are and working with what you've got without fear. Why be afraid? When there is flow, there is no fear. Being defenceless, there is no need to defend anything. Achieving that state of no resistance which I call *defencelessness* requires stripping down our harnesses, shields and defence mechanisms. The only way is to open up to our Higher Self and trust that we can thrive in any circumstance. This state will help us to become aware of our conditioning, habitual patterns, negative self-talk, judgements, emotions and feelings, and we can choose freely what to act upon.

You may experience, at first, that there is much work to be done to get to this state and yet every step is a victory and brings you closer to the state of effortlessness. By detaching from the challenges of our material dimension we can connect better with our spirit. Emotional armour traps us in past events and we project our pain and issues into the morphogenetic field attracting more of the same. Emotional balancing combined with vulnerability lets us deal with the past so we can stay in the present and we can truly experience the meaning of free choice!

EMOTIONS AND CHI

Emotions colour our inner sensations. The broad classification of emotions breaks them into 'pleasant' or 'unpleasant', good or bad, positive or negative. For practical reasons, this is not helpful; it does not give you enough feedback to take appropriate action. Emotions are different from the judgements we make about them, and also different from the actions we take as a result. For emotional balance we can use how we are feeling as a guide to which meridians need balancing – but the biggest discovery to be made is that we may have spent our lives thus far labelling our emotions in a way that does not correspond with reality. A phobia, for example, may be experienced as fear for one person, anxiety and low self-esteem for another. Worries may be labelled as frustration. Another phenomenon is that most emotional states encompass a mix of feelings; by labelling we emphasize only one. Also, there is a difference between the sensations that involve parts of the body and our subjective experience of the moment.

What is important in emotional balance is that, over time, we learn to relinquish false control over the ever-changing scenario we call life. Everything happens in the present; by holding on to something, we shift our awareness from the present to a situation already gone, and keep pulling it back into the present: it controls us and takes us hostage. Some people are always complaining, others are depressed no matter what is going on, others are angry at everyone and yet others are constantly brooding and worrying over details. What do they have in common? They are all living and reliving the past. Whatever presents itself in their lives cannot be appreciated for what it is because of their habitual emotional state.

Emotional balance changes all that; it can be used at any time and any place. Once mastered, it can be accessed any time you are stressed, irritated, upset or worried. It will help you to express what you are feeling in an appropriate way while enabling you to realize that what you are feeling is coloured by the past. Men are better at expressing anger, frustration and irritation, and women are better at expressing grief, sorrow and fear. With emotional balance you have access to the full range of emotions without getting caught up in the turbulence.

Emotional balance means you will no longer project your feelings onto another: 'You make me upset because...' 'You hurt me when you act like that', 'You are making me angry each time you...'. Instead, you will be able to speak from a place of balance: 'I fear that if you say that, it means...' 'I feel anger, when you say...' 'I feel tense and irritated, when...'. The lesson here is that *you can never blame someone else for how you feel!* How you feel is your choice, even if you don't experience it as a choice.

AFFIRMATIONS

By first acknowledging and accepting what you feel and realizing that it is a choice, you can find a more appropriate way of expressing it. Every time you suppress or ignore an emotion, you reject a part of yourself; you are actually telling yourself that you don't really respect yourself.

Affirmations are a way to focus your awareness on what you really want. By simultaneously massaging the meridian-points (see pages 148–61) we open our subconscious mind to the affirmation. Instead of fighting it or creating negative self-talk, the harmony induced will be greater than can be achieved just by using the affirmations alone or just by massaging the emotional balance (EB) points. After a while, positive affirmations will become second nature because the body will link them with the harmony induced by working with the EB points.

Normally positive affirmations cause a lot of resistance because they are alien to us; negative self-talk is the normal pattern for almost everyone. We need to break with all negative affirmations permanently, such as 'My job is terrible' or 'I hate the way I look'. Make positive statements about how you want your life to be; combine these with the Fear Release Points (page 148) and you will be on your way to reprogramming your subconscious mind for success.

Remember always to phrase your affirmation in the *present* tense, for example, 'I am happy' or 'I am feeling good about how

I look' or 'I have everything I need to be happy'. Combine this with visualizing experiencing and enjoying what you want to see manifesting in your life. Make it multi-sensorial; engage in those feelings. Do not use sentences such as 'I will...' or 'I desire...' because your subconscious mind will think these are future goals and will keep them that way.

ACCEPTANCE AND LOVE OF SELF

The most important step to creating a new habitual pattern is *to respect, accept and love yourself.* This is the conditioning that will lead to unconditional happiness. Happiness does not come from health, wealth, beauty, youth or power. Happiness is not something that happens; it is not based on genetics, good fortune or coincidence. It is not the result of any outside event; it is, rather, how we evaluate what happens to us and, on a higher level, how we evaluate our own creation. We should prepare ourselves by accepting and loving all the emotions we create about all the things that we make happen to us. Loving yourself is the fuel of happiness and makes you feel good. It is impossible without self-acceptance and self-approval.

In order to reach this state, we need to train the mind to work for us instead of against us. Our inner critic is programmed to resist change; it is afraid that the unknown is worse than the known. With emotional balancing we can break through the patterns which, in the long run, are self-destructive and will create disease. The key to emotional balance is the focus on what we are feeling.

We will now look at the seven primary emotions which have the biggest impact on our energy flow. All other emotions are connected to these basic seven. We will also review the gateways to balancing these emotions. By conditioning ourselves to deal with these emotions, we will eliminate all tension from the body.

1. FEAR

Fear is the governing emotional condition that drains the *Chi*. Fear comes from imminent threats to our lives. It is based on the idea that we cannot endure a certain situation and may lose what is most precious to us: our life, a loved one, our livelihood, our possessions, our sanity. Fear is the emotion of matter and the most powerful creator of disease.

Element	Water
Organs	Bladder, kidneys
Primary related emotions	Insecurity, indecisiveness
Secondary related emotions	Mistrust, suspicion, despair
Affirmation	'I deeply love and accept myself with my fear and insecurity.'
Primary EB point	At both sides of the breastbone, under the clavicle

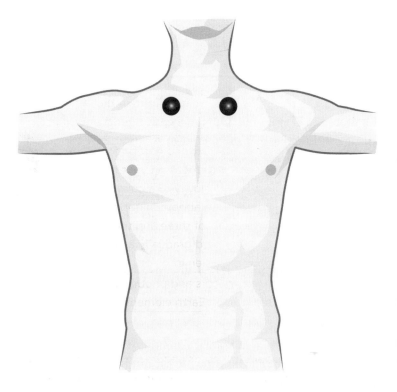

Secondary EB point	At the eyebrows

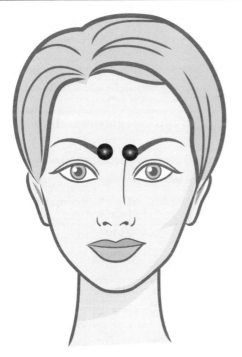

Notes	One of the keys to getting fear under control is to focus on your breathing. Breathe in slowly to a count of seven, pushing the abdomen out; hold your breath for a count of three and then breathe out as slowly and gradually as you can, pulling your abdomen in.
Remarks	Panic attacks and phobias are often related to anxiety (Earth element: *see* Worry)

2. ANGER

Anger is, when suppressed or not appropriately addressed, very damaging to our heart and other vital organs. Anger comes from many different causes: feeling that you have been treated unfairly, not being understood, not getting what you want, feeling insulted. The key is that it does not matter who or what makes us angry; it is an energy that needs to be released and let out of the system. It clouds our vision and logic and makes us take hasty, impulsive decisions.

Element	Wood
Organs	Liver, gallbladder
Primary related emotions	Frustration, irritation
Secondary related emotions	Disappointment, jealousy, fury, bitterness, inability to forgive or let go
Affirmation	'I deeply love and accept myself with my anger and frustration.'
This affirmation, like all others, can be adapted to specific conditions. For example: 'I deeply love and accept myself with my irritation.'	
Primary EB point	This point lies on the right side, approximately halfway along the lower end of the ribcage on the front of the body from the midline to the side.

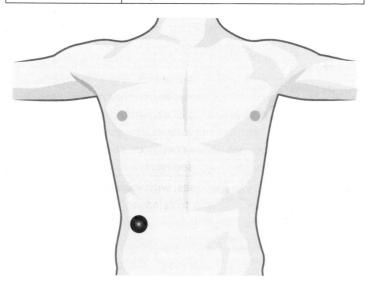

| Secondary EB point | This lies half a finger-width (on the horizontal line) from the corners of the eyes. |

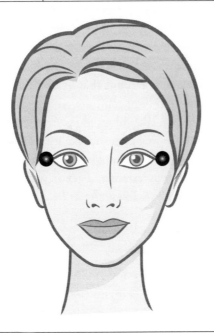

| Notes | When we are angry at someone, we always have to let go of that energy. In order to do this we need to forgive the person who evoked our anger. We also need to forgive ourselves for letting anyone make us angry. As long as a person can make us angry, that means that we are not letting go of something. If someone has the intent to provoke us, it is even easier; we should not waste energy on something like that. For forgiveness: *see* Hurt |
| Remarks | Breathing exercises, with loud screams or sounds, can help to release the energy of anger. Better is physical exercise, running, jumping, using a punching bag, etc. |

3. HURT

Being hurt is one of the most awful feelings and can lead to armouring yourself and feeling inadequate, lonely, guilty, depressed and worthless. It makes you realize you are vulnerable and often taken advantage of. It is an in-between feeling that can go anywhere: withdrawal, denial, confusion, anger, mistrust, fear, etc. This is because hurt resonates most with the heart and with being open and vulnerable. It is a feeling that we can learn to let go of and see that the actions of other people are ways for us to get to know about ourselves. Do we take things too personally? Do we look for ways to grow? How do we handle our reality? Can anyone take our happiness away? Do you love yourself? The only way to deal with hurt is head-on, learn our lessons and get on with our lives. Sharing our intimate feelings can help as long as we take responsibility and not go into victim mode.

Element	Fire
Organs	Heart and small intestine
Primary related emotions	Vulnerability, emotional instability
Secondary related emotions	Hypersensitivity, feeling abandoned, loneliness, suppression of emotions, overexcitement, guilt, shame, disappointment
Affirmation	'I deeply love and accept myself with my feelings of being hurt and forgive myself and [insert the name of the person who has hurt you] for creating this.'
Primary EB point	This point is situated at the inner corner of the cuticle of the little finger on both hands, next to the adjacent finger.

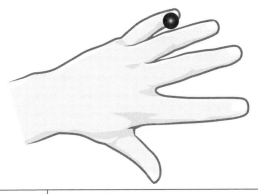

Secondary EB point	With the fists clenched, this lies at the end of the main crease of the palm (left and right hand).

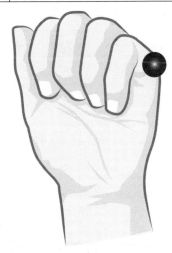

Notes	The power of forgiveness is the most liberating and healing power available to us if we want to let go of the past. *We can never forgive too much!* By forgiving we break our bonds with the past and let go of bad karma. Forgive anyone who has done anything to hurt you.
Remarks	By stimulating the primary point of hurt and forgiving simultaneously we are regenerating our heart and liver and will feel more revitalized.

4. WORRY

This makes us lose a lot of energy and creates tension in the body. It also affects our digestion and metabolism. When we are worried we lose our focus and don't get much done. In the long run this affects our self-esteem. It takes us out of the present. We are more prone to accidents and are distracted easily. By dealing with this effectively, we can accomplish much more and reach our goals with greater ease.

Element	Earth
Organs	Stomach, spleen and pancreas
Primary related emotions	Anxiety, low self-esteem
Secondary related emotions	Dependency, co-dependency, feeling out of control, mistrust, fear of the future, disgust, obsessiveness, neurosis, unhappiness, fear of missing out
Affirmation	'I deeply love and accept myself, also when I am worried, anxious or feel low self-esteem.'
Primary EB points	These points lie in the middle of the bony edge of the eye sockets.

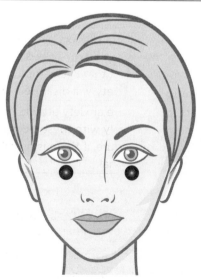

Secondary EB point	This point is the only one on the left side, and is where for women the bra crosses the longitudinal line that is on the side of the body originating exactly from the middle of the armpit.

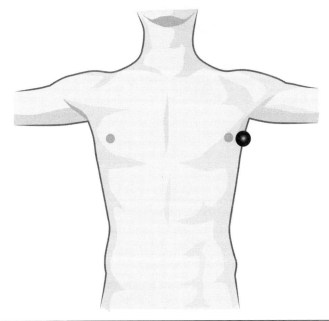

Notes	Every time we are preoccupied and cannot let go of a thought, the primary EB points for worry will help to break that cycle. Also recurrent dreams and anxiety will disappear quickly.
Remarks	Many phobias are anxiety attacks that can be treated effectively with these points. As with any self-help procedure, if there is no relief, consult a health professional.

5. GRIEF

Grief is always related to letting go of a loved one or a cherished possession, and is a very helpful and necessary process. If we were more open to the thought that nothing and no one is ever lost to us, and we understood the workings of the universe, loss would be much easier to bear and accept. It is our attachment that creates the yearning for what we no longer have in our lives. In very traumatic or acutely stressful situations, we may be overwhelmed by strong and intense grief which may be very difficult to let go of and can lead to post-traumatic stress disorder because we have suppressed these emotions. This will lead to a constant fight against the past, and for most people if they don't get help they will not overcome this and may resort to alcohol, drugs or medication to alleviate the symptoms. Because crying alone and dwelling on grief is mostly not enough, we need to open up the flow of the meridians again to restore wellbeing. This is where emotional balancing can be of great help.

Element	Metal
Organs	Lungs, colon
Primary related emotion	Rigidity
Secondary related emotions	Sadness, depression, loss, yearning, desire, loss of faith, hopelessness, inflexibility, defensiveness, holding on to rules, perfectionism, guilt
Primary affirmation	'I deeply love and accept myself with my grief and sense of loss.'
Secondary affirmation	'I deeply love and accept myself with my rigidity and difficulty in letting go.'
Primary EB points	These points lie on the inner side of the cuticle of the thumbs.

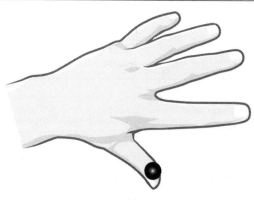

Secondary EB points	These points lie on the index fingers at the side of the thumbs, next to the cuticle.

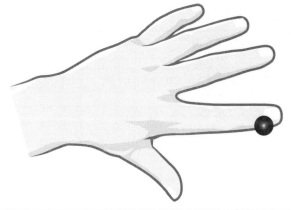

Notes	After grieving we must always restore our Chi. A fast way to do that is to activate all the EB points one by one while repeating the appropriate affirmations.
Remarks	The other patterns locked into the metal element also have to do with holding on to rigidity and perfectionism. These patterns are quite hard to break, but with practice anyone can loosen up and become more flexible.

6. STRESS

Stress is not something we can ignore. Stress is anything that saps energy from our system. Stress has everything to do with how we handle what comes across our path. It has everything to do with our internal processes and nothing to do with external events.

We can deal with stress in a few ways:

1. Resist
2. Suppress our feelings
3. Accept, integrate, release

What we resist will persist, what we suppress will haunt us forever. So the best way is to make stress disappear into thin **AIR**: act upon what we can change and control; **i**ntegrate by accepting what we cannot change or control; **r**elease any tension that inhibits free flow.

Element	Fire
Organs	Immuno-endocrinal system (Governor and Conception Vessel)
Primary related emotion	Suppression of emotions
Secondary related emotions	Nostalgia, confusion, repression of anger, feelings of emptiness, insecurity, problems with concentration and memory
Primary affirmation	'I deeply love and accept myself with my stress.'
Secondary affirmation	'I deeply love and accept myself even when I suppress my emotions.'
Primary EB point	This point is at the junction of the upper third and lower two-thirds of a line joining the nose and middle of the upper lip.

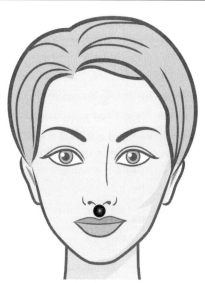

Secondary EB point	This point is at the junction of the upper third and lower two-thirds of a line joining the middle of the upper lip and the chin.

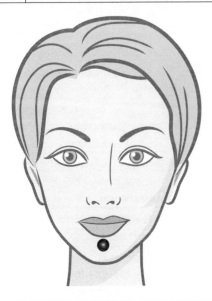

Notes	Nostalgia is reliving the past; we are not in the present and we are stuck in a daydreaming mode that will take away the possibility of dealing with our karma. We need to let go of what could have been and create what we really want now.
Remarks	Learning to deal with stress is one of the most helpful skills we can have in our modern lives. Staying calm and centred amidst the turmoil is the key for health and longevity.

7. OVEREXCITEMENT

Overexcitement and emotional instability are not far from each other. In the search for pleasure and excitement we can get disconnected from feeling. By tuning in to the feelings inside we can get connected again. By placing a hand over our forehead we connect the left- and right-brain reflex areas; this will calm us down and help integrate our inner turbulence, especially when we perform deep abdominal breathing and focus on 'letting go' with each exhalation. Repeat these soothing words (the primary affirmation) for as long as needed to reclaim your emotional balance.

Element	Fire
Organs	Pericardium and Triple Burner (neuro-endocrine system)
Primary related emotions	Repressed sexuality
Secondary related emotions	Changing moods, paranoia, indecisiveness, confusion, loss of libido, frigidity, impotence, exhaustion, shock, acute trauma
Primary affirmation	'I am feeling balanced and am able to deal with all my challenges, however big, gracefully.'
Secondary affirmation	'I deeply feel the love for myself and accept my suppressed feelings about my sexuality.'
Primary EB point	On the top of either hand, midway between the bottom-most knuckles and the wrist; in the valley between the third and little finger

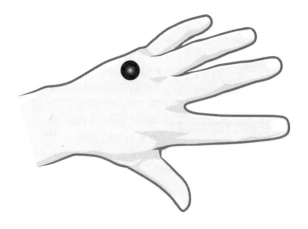

Secondary EB points	On the middle fingers of both hands, next to the corner of the cuticle on the thumb side

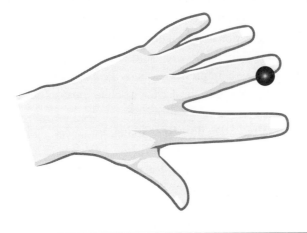

Notes	There are many ways and reasons to suppress our sexuality that are not directly related to sex. Sexuality is about feminine and masculine qualities in both men and women. Men tend to suppress their feminine side and live more in denial. By not acknowledging their most intimate feelings they are repressing their sexuality. They can also repress their masculine side by not being assertive. Women tend to suppress their masculine, assertive side by not appropriately dealing with anger.
Remarks	Neurological instability is very common these days. The sensory input can become too much and there is not enough opportunity to release 'pent-up' emotions; we become hyper and overexcited. The other side is that we can get drained and become exhausted. In the fast-changing world in which we are living, the traditional male–female roles may become blurred – with repressed emotions as the consequence.

SUMMARY

What I have presented in this chapter are the basics for emotional balancing, one of the fastest-working therapies known in managing the emotions. I have been teaching this technique to health professionals throughout Europe, who use it in their daily practice. The results are astounding. I also teach a version to laypeople, with impressive results. People have succeeded in overcoming alcoholism, headaches, phobias, post-traumatic stress, chronic fatigue syndrome, allergies, nightmares, shyness, fear of public speaking, addiction to smoking and more. Relationships and marriages have been saved. In the following chapters I will introduce additional tools and a protocol for using EB in your daily life.

The seven primary emotions are the main stressors to our system that we need to learn how to handle: fear, anger, hurt, grief, worry, stress and overexcitement. In the chapters to come we will start cleaning up all your major emotional traumas – so quickly that you will be wondering why all psychologists and doctors don't use these methods.

I will end this chapter with this thought (from nineteenth-century French poet and dramatist Edmond Rostand); see if you can make a habit of saying it to yourself every day while looking in the mirror: *I love you more than yesterday and less than tomorrow.*

CHAPTER 9

EMOTIONAL REVERSAL

If I told you that I will reveal to you the biggest secret I've uncovered in healing, which works for 99 per cent of the people who use it, and that I know that most of you, reading this, do *not* use it, would you believe me? Would you use it if you knew it could change your life exponentially for the better and that you would have more fun, more success and longevity with good health and less stress, fewer frustrations, worries and fears?

Why do you suppose most people sabotage themselves? Why do most people procrastinate? Why don't most people follow through on their New Year's resolutions? Why do most people say they want to be happy, yet do everything to destroy their relationships and be miserable? Why do people severely harm their bodies and health? Why do most people ignore doctors' orders? Why do more than 95 per cent of dieters gain the weight back plus a bit more? Why do we choose laziness, lies, half-truths, negligence, ignorance, denial or suppression when we could have it all? Whom can we blame for our self-sabotage and failure?

CASE STUDY: SELF-SABOTAGE

John was a boy of 14; he was very good at judo. According to his *sensei* (teacher), John was the best talent he had seen in all of his 30-plus years of expertise in judo. John came to see me after his parents saw me on TV and heard that I had also been a European judo champion many years before and was now coaching some world-champion athletes on an emotional and mental level, with great success. John had never won first prize. All the matches leading up to the final he would win effortlessly, but when it came to the final he would lose.

I tested John for emotional blocks. When he said, 'I want to be a champion' his muscles tested weak, indicating an incongruence. An incongruence is when you consciously want something but subconsciously you have reasons to fear that outcome, or you may believe that you do not deserve it, or that it is impossible or unrealistic. When it comes to the mind and subconscious mind, if one wants to go right and the other left, you have a big problem. In the long run, the subconscious mind will win most of the time (causing, if necessary, stress, distractions and detours). The conscious mind is you; what you want or desire. In this chapter you will learn how to synchronize the conscious and subconscious mind and let them work together for you.

I told John, 'A part of you is afraid of being a champion. Let's dig deeper and find out how this came about, and then we can do something about it!' John was visibly excited; this problem had been embarrassing him for so long and he was eager to get over it and trample his reputation for being number two. As a matter of fact he was due to participate the following week in the selections for the national team. He had even read my book, *You Are a Champion*, in which I describe the emotional and mental techniques that helped me become undefeated European champion in martial arts for seven years.

What I found with muscle-testing was that there had been some sort of incident shortly after John's birth. This incident I could not define exactly; it came out that it was something the doctor had said. I looked at John's mother and asked her if anything had happened. She told me that John was her first-born. The delivery had been very painful and the doctor had used forceps to get John out. She remembered that the doctor made a remark along the lines of: 'That's always the problem with the first one; they cause the most pain and trouble.' She also remembered that she had said a 'rude word' when the doctor was stitching her up. She said, 'I was so tired and he was a little brusque and not compassionate at all, and they would not give Johnny to me straightaway, so I was a little bit irritated.'

The little newborn had picked all of this up and associated being 'the first one' with causing his mother pain, and had subconsciously decided never to be first again. When I tested John on the following statement: 'I do not want to be first, because that causes pain to my mother,' his muscles were strong, indicating that, for his subconscious mind, this was true.

After the session John was very excited; he felt ready and wanted the match to be the next day. A week later they rang me up late in the morning; first his mother was on the phone to tell me that John had won. Then I spoke to John himself, who was so excited he could barely speak. He gave me a full report on how he'd defeated a long-time rival, who had been national champion for three years running. His feeling that something was holding him back had disappeared, as if by magic.

John's story has many variations in daily life: we want to have a happy and great relationship with our partner, yet we are locked into unproductive patterns which keep us apart emotionally and eventually lead to pain, abuse, escape in alcohol, cigarettes or food, and relationship breakdown.

CASE STUDY: CAN'T QUIT SMOKING

I was presenting a lecture on emotional balance to a crowd of 600 people. After my general introduction, it was time for a demonstration. I asked for a volunteer with an issue that was not too complicated, just to keep it simple. Around 10 people put up their hands; I selected a young woman in her thirties for no other reason than I felt it was the right thing to do. In these selections I always follow my intuition, and always someone comes up who is very helpful in illustrating my point.

This woman's name was Joan and her problem was that she'd just about quit smoking – but could not give up completely and still smoked one cigarette a day. She hated herself for this and had tried hypnosis, acupuncture and nicotine chewing gum, to no avail. I explained to her that addictions are always predominantly mental/emotional and almost never chemically-induced, and that when we stop an addiction with willpower or with the use of aids such as nicotine patches, chewing gums or herbs, we are not addressing the underlying subconscious causes. I also explained that behind each addiction there is a positive intent either to cover up some emotional wound, self-harm because of negative beliefs or a hidden quest for spirituality. The latter we see more with mind-altering drugs, where people try to take a short cut to the path to enlightenment.

I asked Joan, 'What does this one cigarette give you?' She said, 'It gives me the feeling of personal space, something just for me. I run around all day keeping the house clean and doing stuff for the children and my husband; this is like quality time for me!' She explained that she had developed a whole routine around smoking her cigarette. She would turn on classical music, get herself a glass of wine and sit down in her favourite chair and put her feet up and smoke. I asked her why she wanted to let go of that cigarette, and she told me that despite what the cigarette did for her, she also had the fear that it would kill her. Her father had been a chain-smoker and had developed lung cancer and suffered for four years before he'd passed away. She had been with him when he died.

Joan had a love-hate relationship with her cigarette: on the one hand it gave her tremendous pleasure, and on the other she associated pain, suffering and death with it. After her cigarette she would always feel overwhelmed by guilt, low self-esteem and sadness. So it seemed like a clear-cut case.

I had already explained to my audience that night that, strangely enough, in my research I had found that the big traumas were never behind the most neurotic or compulsive or self-sabotaging behaviours. What I had found, testing thousands of patients, was that underlying most cases of post-traumatic suffering were minor incidents in the past that led to an inability to cope with the big incidents or traumas in our lives. Also that sometimes we come into this world with some 'short-circuit' in our cell-memory, either from previous lives or previous generations.

So I started to check Joan on which emotions were holding her back from letting go of that last cigarette. There were five emotions: sadness, fear, insecurity, suppression of sexuality and frustration. Then I went on to check what had caused her to hold on to these emotions. It had something to do with an incident when she was three years old. The details that came out were: she had been home completely absorbed in playing; her mother had been in the kitchen cooking. She'd heard a noise like something falling; when she went to investigate she'd found her mum unconscious on the kitchen floor. She'd panicked, screamed and run outside to get the neighbours. They were not at home. She was completely frustrated and kept pressing the doorbell, crying and screaming. A postman coming along found her, brought her back home and called the ambulance. Everything worked out fine: the mother had anaemia and low blood pressure, but recovered completely. Joan associated 'having time for herself' with this painful incident. The only emotion that was not part of that incident was her suppressed sexuality. That we traced back to around her fourth month in the womb, when her parents had had the first sonogram. When the technician told her parents she was a girl, her father said, 'Damn, I had hoped for a boy!' Somehow, she'd either picked up on that or the disappointment behind it.

Joan told the audience that now she understood why she had been a tomboy and why she hated all the traditional 'woman's' chores. That is why she attached so much value to her 'quality time', to recharging emotionally after all the chores associated with being a woman. With her father's disappointment she had linked fear of the outside world, insecurity and frustration. Her whole life she had been trying to prove herself, and had felt insecure and lacking in self-esteem. She'd picked up smoking in her early teens to 'belong' and for the first time she was accepted in a group. After her father died she quit smoking except for that last cigarette. What finally came out was that she felt guilty for the relief she had felt when her father had died: she no longer had to prove that she was worthy of his love. Subconsciously, that last cigarette was her last connection with her father, her last effort to connect to him. When she said, 'Quitting this last cigarette means losing contact with my father,' her muscles were testing very strong!

Once we integrated the emotions and her subconscious mind let go of them, she tested weak on that statement, indicating she had let go of that subconscious belief. She felt a surge of emotion coming through, and she cried. The audience, which had been silent during all the time it took to unravel this story, started to applaud and she got a standing ovation for her story. You could feel the empathy of the audience for her.

I never spoke to Joan again, but I am sure that she no longer smokes. I did receive some feedback from at least 10 people who wrote to me after that session to tell me they had spontaneously quit smoking from then on.

With this case study one can see that something as simple as one cigarette can get quite complicated – and that it is not about willpower or mental focus. Willpower is not good or bad, but when we use it to suppress our emotions, we create negative energy that will cost us dearly, sooner or later.

HOW EMOTIONAL REVERSAL WORKS

Emotional reversal is when we want something and at the same time our subconscious mind is not aligned with it. This will cause considerable amount of stress in the body, which can be measured with biofeedback equipment, a voice-stress analyzer or with simple muscle-testing. When you say something that is not congruent with your subconscious mind, a muscle that is normally strong will immediately lose its strength and test weak. This happens when you are thinking about your goals. Every time we think about our goals, if we are not congruent, we lose some vital life-force.

Subconscious Programming

Our subconscious is programmed just as computer software is programmed. This concept comes from the field known as cognitive science and is called *functionalism*. Functionalism states that intelligent procedures undertaken in order to achieve a common outcome will reflect the same or similar underlying processes. Functionalism concludes, therefore, that the subconscious mind is to a person what a software program is to a computer's hardware. We do not need to know anything about how the brain functions on a biological level in order to program it.

The only problem with cognitive science is that it leaves out the emotions. By working with the emotions we can bypass the resistance caused by our unresolved issues, which otherwise will eventually lead to failure.

The subconscious mind is especially suited to help us achieve what we want. It is like an automatic pilot: it will bring us to whatever destiny we have requested. It will not settle for anything less than success – but if success for you means staying in your comfort zone, even if you are miserable, it will find all the ways possible to help you feel miserable. If your goal, however, is to be happy, it will set you on course. So let's look at your 'successes' now; check if there is an area where you can recognize being successful in achieving what you *don't* want.

Health

Pain, accidents, surgery (to remove gallbladder, tonsils, appendix, stomach, fibroid tumours, cancer, polyps and other growths), broken bones, scars, premature ageing, a weak immune system, autoimmune diseases, diabetes, high blood pressure, infections, chronic fatigue syndrome, allergies, stiffness, loss of hearing or vision, etc. – the list can go on forever. You should look closely at this area of your life if you've had chronic conditions, operations and/or have been to the doctor's surgery more often than you can remember. If you are not enjoying vibrant health, you are probably sabotaging yourself in this area. If you are smoking, drinking more than two drinks a day, overweight by more than 12 pounds, do not exercise and have never attempted meditation, yoga, Tai Chi or Qigong, you are probably emotionally reversed on health.

Relationships

Attracting people who make you miserable is a clue that you are emotionally reversed in this area of life. Sometimes referred to as *toxic people*, in my philosophy there are no toxic people as such. The degree to which a person stresses you (*is toxic to you*) is the same as the degree to which you allow him or her to stress you (*be toxic to you*). If you work on changing yourself, you will see that two things happen:

1.   **You will attract other types of people into your life.**
2.   **The *toxic people* will either not be toxic to you anymore or they will change, too.**

People who stress you are those who annoy you, don't support you, are demanding, smothering, mothering, abusive, don't pay attention to you, always criticize you, are unloving or take you for granted. If you feel miserable on a regular basis and think you have no choice but to settle for what you've got, that you don't deserve to be happy or that life is just cruel like that, then you are probably emotionally reversed in this area.

Finances

Your pay cheque does not last you the whole month, you juggle payments, cannot save or invest, cannot hold down a job. There is never enough money, you give it away to others without keeping enough for yourself, you buy lottery tickets hoping to hit the big one.

Money problems are rampant in our society; many people live from payday to payday and have no way out. Others work two or more jobs to make ends meet, while others with good jobs still live above their means. Most people have a love–hate relationship with money. There are many reasons to self-sabotage in this area when in your subconscious mind you believe that money is the root of all evil, money never makes anyone happy and many other incongruities.

Money represents energy; by not having enough money, which in turn stresses you and saps more energy, you are in a vicious cycle that can only change when your subconscious programming about money is altered.

TOTAL EMOTIONAL REVERSAL (TER)

This is where subconsciously you are programmed to fail on *all* levels of life. Your relationship does not work, you have financial stress, health problems and there is no end in sight. You may have been to motivational seminars (I call these 'temporary feel-good sessions'), psychologists and medical doctors; you may have tried meditation and may have read self-help books and listened to endless self-help tapes – all with only temporary results or none. Your conclusions are somewhere along the lines of: 'Life is tough, I am a failure, I have no talents, I am not born for luck, I can't do anything right, I am only doing this because there is nothing else.' You probably procrastinate most of the time and have a lot of self-pity. These are all part of being massively emotionally reversed.

Time to Journal

How Do You Feel?

By now you should have a pretty good picture of where you are sabotaging yourself. Do not feel depressed if it is in more than one area, or even all of them; that is fairly common, and happily the solution is easy and effective. Answer the following questions as honestly as you can and make notes in your journal, because all of this is about to change dramatically in your life:

171

- How do you feel about yourself?
- Are you comfortable saying: 'I am extremely successful!'?
- What is going on in your life that you feel good about?
- What are the things that frustrate you, irritate you or give you stress?
- Do you like what you are doing most of the time?
- Do you wake up eager and hungry to get going?
- How are your finances? Do you feel happy with what you have?
- How are your relationships (partner, children, friends, family)?
- Do you have many stressful relationships?
- What were your youth and your childhood like?
- When you think of your parents, do you feel happy or peaceful?
- Do you feel happy, healthy and lucky?

If any of these questions makes you feel uncomfortable or causes you stress, then we are looking at some issues that are robbing you of life-force. You may not be in touch with your feelings or in denial; that is definitely an area to work on, too. Emotional reversal results in a lot of pain, suffering, misery and feelings of inadequacy.

Keywords

Three of the keywords that you will hear from people who are emotionally reversed are: 'should', 'try' and 'maybe'. They say things like, 'I should take better care of my health,' 'I should exercise,' 'I will try to quit smoking,' 'Maybe I will start dieting tomorrow.'

Excuses Are Proof of Reversal

Others have excuses, and say things like:

'I do not have enough willpower.'
'I am the way I am; I am not perfect.'
'I am too lazy; I've always been like this.'

'We all have to die of something.'

'I don't feel that I will ever be happy, no matter what I do.'

Three Little Words that Indicate Reversal

Here are the problems with the three words that are commonly used with emotionally reversed people.

1. Maybe

When we say *maybe*, we do not commit to something; we leave the door wide open *not* to do what we intended to do. We make it really easy on ourselves so we cannot fail. This is self-defeat before we've even started, and seldom leads to success. *Maybe* is a stressful word for the subconscious mind, and in itself takes away any goal-setting for our mind. No action will be taken if we have other priorities.

2. Try

Try is very similar. You cannot *try* to do anything and be successful. *Trying* means not taking action in the world, but only in your mind. Let's take an easy example; *try* to read the next sentence: *if you are reading this sentence, you are not trying – go back and try to read it again!* You see, if you *try* to do something and do it, you are not *trying* anymore, you are doing. You cannot *try* to do something and do it; that is impossible. So do yourself a big favour and ban *try* completely from your vocabulary; it's another word that causes stress to your subconscious mind. Delete it permanently, and if you catch yourself saying it, replace it with: '*I will do my best*' or '*I will do everything in my power to make this happen.*'

3. Should

Let's look at the mother of all bad words: *should*. *Should* is probably the worst of this trio, because every time we say *should*, we 'shoot' ourselves in the foot. The word *should* implies we are at fault, we are inadequate, or we were inadequate, or we will be inadequate in the future. It confirms we are inadequate in being who we are. *Should* is better replaced by *could*, as this gives us more positive options.

Procrastination and Resistance

Every time we use *should*, *maybe* or *try*, we are sabotaging ourselves and not being truthful to ourselves; we are not making real choices and instead we open the door wide for sabotage and procrastination to come in. When we resist something this is based on the fact that we are not congruent with what we think we want to do, could do or are doing.

Self-image Lies at the Heart of Self-sabotage

Under all of this is our negative self-image that we are not good enough. In other words, we believe that we are not lovable and we reject ourselves, and thus sabotage our own goals and objectives. That is why 'positive thinking' and affirmations cannot work when they are inconsistent with our self-image. A negative self-image comes from how we interpret the input we've received in the past. For example, if a parent says, 'I do not like the way you are behaving,' it is very difficult for the child to make a distinction between behaviour and identity. So, now the child thinks he is not a lovable person because his parent dislikes him. That becomes his reality. Our present self-image and the resulting self-esteem come out of what we have experienced (our emotional reality) rather than what actually happened. So now we have to change that emotional reality by taking away the negative charge of the past emotional reality. We have to give a new meaning to our past and thus change the experience in the now.

The secret to changing your life is not reading this book, but *experiencing* this book by applying its information to your reality. The first step is to identify the issues in your life that need work. Make note of that. The second step is to work on yourself by undertaking certain exercises. You need around three to four weeks to start experiencing real change in your life. Any expectations for faster results are not realistic – though that's not to say you won't see results more quickly than this. Reserve all judgement for a minimum of three weeks; that's how long it takes to change a negative self-image and break through emotional reversal and sabotage.

Changing a negative self-image into an empowering self-image will mean the difference between success and failure, honesty and dishonesty, love and fear, misery and happiness. It can help you rescue a marriage that is going downhill, recharge your life and career, transform you from victim to victor. Creating an empowering self-image means the difference between emotional freedom and being an emotional hostage.

Stopping Self-sabotage

Whether we know it or not, we have a subconscious image of ourselves; this is a fully detailed concept of who you believe you are. This image is the end result of all the programming and conditioning you've endured in this lifetime and, if you are open to the idea, many previous lifetimes. Our karma and duty are to 'update our files' and 'delete from our software' all data which, with our current consciousness and knowledge, no longer serve us. If you are reading this book, you know that we are unlimited beings. All of our limitations come from unresolved issues that we have chosen to hold on to. We have chosen to believe the lies that our parents, peers, teachers and other so-called authorities told us. We have been misled to be sheep, while in reality we are born to be lions. We have learned to bleat instead of roar. We have bought into the illusion of material reality by being a five-sensed person instead of multi-sensorial. We have chosen to believe that we are not successful, not lovable, not worthy, not deserving and not attractive. We have succeeded in limiting ourselves to the lower levels of happiness instead of unconditional happiness. We have not let go of our humiliations, failures and perceived rejection by others. We have forgotten that we are creators of our own destiny and that we all are immortal, unlimited spirits coming from the Source of love, here on Earth by choice to find ways of transcending the self-imposed limitations of the flesh. So now that you are completely aware of the magnificent being trapped inside, you can move on to the next stage of awareness and start creating the kind of self-image that will be your automatic pilot for success, health, longevity and happiness.

Consistency

All that you do, feel or think is always consistent with your self-image. You are programmed to be a certain way, whether you like it or not, so you will behave in a way consistent with that. If you are emotionally programmed for failure, you will find one way after another to stay consistent with your 'failure-orientated' personality. You will sabotage your success in any way you can. An example is getting stuck in a traffic jam on the way to an important meeting. You might think that a traffic jam is something beyond your control, especially when it happens unexpectedly, but if your self-image is 'victim', you will attract (read: create) situations in your life that will bear out exactly what you believe. Understanding the fact that we are living biological transmitters and receivers, we can come to the realization that we are magnets to people and situations that will be consistent with our self-image. We create our own self-fulfilling prophecies: if you don't feel attractive, you will create that reality and find confirmation for your belief. It goes even further than this: if you don't believe you are lovable, your brain will filter out all messages that say otherwise.

At one of my seminars, one of the participants came up to ask for my personal help. Hannah's problem was that she thought that nobody loved her, including her husband and her children. When I asked her how come she'd married someone who did not love her, she said, 'Everybody loves me in the beginning, but they lose interest after a while!' I got her permission to bring her on stage in front of the audience, so everyone could learn from her situation. Her husband was also asked on stage. I asked him to tell her that he loved her. Immediately her muscles went weak – an indication that she was being stressed by this statement. Then I asked her husband just to look at her lovingly and connect with his love inside for her. Again she immediately was stressed. Then I asked him to tell her that he did *not* love her. Now she was strong, meaning that her subconscious mind accepted that message and did not resist that. Then I asked him to look as if he were angry and upset with her and not say anything; she was also comfortable with this (indicated by muscle strength). In other words, she was emotionally reversed on being loved.

What I learned was that, when she was around three or four, her sister was born and all the attention went to her. Hannah withdrew herself as much as she could, because she thought her father loved her sister more than he loved her. She also stopped sitting on her father's lap and refused to be cuddled. Her father, for his part, felt rejected by Hannah and paid more attention to her sister. Thus Hannah locked in emotions of bitterness, jealousy, low self-esteem, resentment and grief.

I did a forgiveness session with her, to help her forgive her sister and her father. After that, she was no longer emotionally reversed. This had a great impact on her marriage and life. She is now more self-confident and assertive.

It is important that we seek always to affirm a positive self-image and thus make it stronger. I have seen many miraculous changes in self-confidence, career, relationship or health when a client succeeds in creating an empowering self-image.

Fear and Acceptance

Our self-image leads to emotional reversal because any time we want something that is not consistent with our self-image, we immediately trigger fear in ourselves. This fear comes from wanting something that is 'not good for us' because it is inconsistent with our self-image. So, if you want to be rich but you have a self-image of not being worthy of wealth, your subconscious mind will find ways to make being rich scary. You will lose friends, or people will only like you because of your money. If you have money, 'they' will try to steal it from you. Many more reasons will come up, and no sane person would want to be rich under those conditions.

How does this apply to something like health? Health may be associated with responsibilities, with having to work, not getting attention, always having to be strong. Disease may be more pleasurable in some ways: it may mean we get attention, love, respect, care, admiration. If as a child you got attention mainly when you were poorly, and you attached pleasure to not going to school, you might have subconsciously created the image that being sick is fun and being healthy is bad.

You might be thinking, *OK, I can understand that this is possible with wealth and health, but how can anyone want to be miserable and not happy?* Yet even being happy can be associated with unpleasant feelings. You might feel that being happy is wrong when there are still so many people suffering in the world. Being happy can therefore actually make you feel guilty. You might believe you don't really deserve to be happy because you are a bad person. You might believe that being happy means not showing empathy or respect to others. Some people have associated so much pain with being happy that they cannot enjoy themselves or experience pleasure.

Psychologist Dr Janet Hranicky has studied the personalities of hundreds of cancer patients and has found that many of them have these negative associations with happiness. She calls this 'pleasure-freeze'. In other words, we can fear what we want when we subconsciously believe it does not fit the image we have of ourselves. One of the techniques we will use teaches us to accept that we may never be happy, healthy or successful. Nobody wants to embrace this, but by accepting that we may never get what we want, we actually take away the self-sabotage that we'd otherwise face when we set out for our goals. If you accept failure as a possibility, it will no longer stress you and you can use the energy you might have wasted on fear to create success. 'I accept and love myself even if I fail' is the answer to changing fear into power. We will get more into this later.

Self-image Is Reprogrammable

The good news is that anyone at any age can change their self-image and thus create peace of mind. This works on the cause and not the symptoms. The symptoms are failure, disease, misery and poverty; the cause is a disempowering self-image. Emotional balance is only achievable if we start with causes. 'Positive thinking' alone is not good enough without changing our self-image. We need to create a self-image that is consistent with our goals, values and commitments.

So the question to ask yourself is simple: 'What kind of self-image do I need to have to achieve what I want in life?' To create a great life you need to have a supporting self-image that is congruent with your beliefs. You must be able to believe in you. Therefore, you have to reprogram your subconscious mind with the 'success' software of your choosing. This will lead to new habits of thinking, imagining and feeling that will be consistent with your new self-image.

Even total emotional reversal can be fixed very simply by using a few affirmations while simultaneously treating some EB points. We will go over this technique at the end of this chapter. The real problem is *not loving ourselves enough*. We feel we are not good enough, not deserving, not worthy. This is all nonsense, and it is time for drastic change and a new life.

SPECIFIC EMOTIONAL REVERSAL (SER)

This is also a means of sabotaging what we really want, but it is not as broad as total emotional reversal. We may be totally congruent with being happy, healthy and successful and still sabotage ourselves in some specific areas of life. Where total emotional reversal leads to a life full of depression, failure and bad health, SER will affect us only in specific areas. We may be very successful in our careers and making a good living, while totally sabotaging another area such as our relationships, health or spiritual growth. We might be very successful in areas such as marriage and health while chronically messing up our finances. Sometimes it looks like simple bad luck – but luck has nothing to do with it. The following story will give you an idea of how this works in real life.

I met Joseph on a plane flying from Amsterdam to Atlanta; I was returning after two weeks of an intensive itinerary with back-to-back seminars and lectures in Italy and the Netherlands. After napping for an hour or so on the flight, I was woken up to have lunch. Next to me, Joseph was not eating; he stared ahead with an empty look in his eyes. He was a good-looking young man in his mid-twenties. I asked him if something was wrong with the food. He said, 'No, I am just not feeling well. Things are not going right for me.' I sympathized, so started to ask questions to see if I could be of any help. His story was remarkable. He was 24 years old and his parents had died in a car accident when he'd been just eight. By a twist of fate they'd left him home that night, despite his very strong vocal requests for them to stay at home with him. They persisted and he had to stay with the live-in maid. His parents were quite rich and left him around $5 million in a trust fund plus some real estate worth another $4 million. When he turned 18, John was free to invest the money any way he wanted. He'd consulted a reputable financial advisor and invested his money in the stock market. Soon after he'd invested his money, the stock market crashed and he'd lost $2 million overnight. He took all his money out and went to Switzerland to invest it in real estate. Just over a year later he lost another million dollars and had only $2 million left. Following the advice of new financial advisors, he invested some of his money in racehorses and in a very well-established restaurant. Here he lost half of his money and, in a last effort to see what he could do, he had flown to Amsterdam to talk to one of the most reputable and consistently successful investment groups. He was depressed because they'd told him it would take at least eight to 10 years to recover his losses. He was thinking of selling all his real estate, even though the market was a buyer's market and he would not get the best price. He believed that he was born to bad luck; first he'd lost his parents and now he was on his way to losing all of his money.

I told him that I was doing research on how the subconscious mind is a built-in automatic pilot leading us to our subconscious beliefs, and that I believed it was reprogrammable. I told him that I would like to help him and that I expected that in his case it would cost him, in the worst-case scenario, only 20 to 30 minutes. He had nothing to lose and we were going to be stuck on the plane for the next six hours anyway, so I started to probe his subconscious mind with muscle-testing. He tested strong on the following statements:

'I want to be healthy.'
'I want to be successful.'

He tested weak on the following statements:

'I want to make money.'
'I want to be lucky.'
'I want to be happy.'

Conversely, he was also strong on the following statements (meaning they were true for him):

'I want to lose all my money.'
'I want to have bad luck.'
'I want to be miserable.'

Now I had Joseph's full attention and he was totally blown away by the outcome of this simple test. 'What's going on? How is this possible?' he asked, completely confused. 'Let's look deeper for the cause of this,' was my answer, and we continued testing. The flight attendant was walking by frequently, staring at the two men performing some strange-looking ritual. When I muscle-test someone, I have them form a so-called O-ring by connecting the tip of the thumb on one hand with the tip of either the index, ring or middle finger of the same hand. I then use both of my hands to test the strength of this 'O-ring' as the person I am testing says the statements I propose. Obviously this looks quite bizarre to any unsuspecting onlooker!

181

I started to check which emotions where unresolved in relation to Joseph's wanting to be financially successful and happy. The following came up: guilt, grief, abandonment, low self-esteem and being unable to forgive. These had not been resolved after his parents had died. What had happened is that he blamed himself for not getting them to stop at home with him; he felt that he was guilty of their deaths and that he did not deserve to inherit their money. He was very unforgiving toward himself and felt abandoned by God, and that caused his low self-esteem and grief.

Subconscious Mind and the Morphogenetic Field

From this story we can learn that the subconscious mind is able to access data we are not aware of. Joseph selected financial advisors with good reputations, whose advice caused him to lose money. It almost seems like the advisors were part of a cosmic conspiracy to help Joseph reach his goal: to get rid of his money. The other way to look at it is that Joseph's subconscious mind had the magic ability to influence real estate values in such a way that his properties lost value, to make winning racehorses lose, or to make loyal customers come less frequently to a restaurant. The third possibility is that both things happened simultaneously: on the one hand being clairvoyant and knowing how to lose money on investments, and on the other to influence the world so it will give you what you want. Of course a fourth possibility would be that this was all coincidence and had nothing to do with Joseph. Some people would like to believe this because they are scared of the idea that our subconscious is powerful and will work relentlessly to achieve our subconscious goals. This is an incredible *success mechanism*, unparalleled by anything we can think of. Yes, there is a *cosmic conspiracy* going on; that is where all collective consciousness meets to create the circumstances that will serve the karma of everyone. So, either we take responsibility and start making use of it, or we keep ignoring it and believe we are victims or just plain lucky or unlucky when things go well or badly.

CASE STUDY: SPECIFIC EMOTIONAL REVERSAL

Paul was uncomfortable with what he had just told me, and stared down at his feet. Lily, his fiancée, seemed comfortable with the situation and looked at me as if I were some kind of judge and should decide whose side I was on. Paul had just told me that he and Lily had been dating for two years and that he always had to push her to have sex. During intercourse she would just lie on her back and allow him to use her, but would not participate or enjoy any of it. He was 26, she was 27. Both said they loved each other and wanted to continue the relationship; it was just that Lily did not like sex and would participate just to please Paul.

Paul had seen me on TV and had arranged the appointment. 'There must be a reason why Lily has such an aversion to sex,' I said. 'I will test her and we will find out more, but before I do, I would like to ask Lily: were you ever molested, raped, sexually or physically abused or a victim of incest?' She said no. The only other symptom that she had was that she had stopped menstruating two years before. She had always had a very irregular menstrual cycle. For six to seven years she would have her period only four times a year. I started to test her for emotional reversal and she was congruent with the following statements (indicating that her subconscious mind agreed!):

'I want to be healthy, happy and successful.'
'I want to have a good relationship.'

She was incongruent with the following statements (indicating that her subconscious mind did not agree):

'I want to be able to enjoy sex.'
'I want to have sex with Paul.'

She was congruent with the following:

'I want to stop having sex with Paul.'
'I want to be miserable having sex.'

183

Both Paul and Lucy were completely amazed by what they were seeing and hearing. The emotions that came up were: grief, shame, despair, sadness, hurt, vulnerability, guilt and disgust. Something had happened when Lucy was 18 that was shocking to her and had caused the suppression of these emotions. I asked her if she knew what had happened nine years before. She immediately started to cry and could not stop for the next five minutes. Then she started to tell her story in bits and pieces.

When she was 18, she became pregnant. Her boyfriend was a schoolmate, also 18, with whom she was in love. She had wanted to keep the baby, but her parents had reacted very negatively, telling her, 'How can you do this to us? You should be ashamed.' They forced Lucy, against her will, to have an abortion. She did not want to because she believed it was murder and she wanted to have the baby. Her parents insisted. When she came home from the clinic, they had bought cake and champagne to celebrate the 'happy ending'. She had fled upstairs to her room to cry and prayed to God: 'Don't ever let this happen again; next time I will kill myself!'

So, Lucy's *subconscious success mechanism* went to work; after that trauma she started to have irregular periods and then none at all. She broke up with that boyfriend and did not date for five years until she'd met Paul three years before. Then she'd discovered that, although she loved Paul, she did not enjoy having sex. She had suppressed all the information about the abortion completely and never thought of it anymore, until now.

We worked on letting go of her emotions and did a forgiveness session to forgive her parents for being so insensitive and for forcing her to have an abortion. What happened afterwards was the closest thing to a miracle one can get. Lucy called one week later to say that she had had six passionate days and nights with Paul and that she was worried about Paul keeping up with her sexual appetite. 'By the way,' she said, 'this morning I got my period!' What the specialists could not do with chemical hormones, her mind had fixed easily and naturally.

The most beautiful thing is that these cases are not rare or uncommon; they happen every day in the lives of people who are using emotional balance to address their turbulence. Everyday people and health professionals are using this method all the time. My wish is that this book spreads the word about these tools to millions more worldwide.

PARTIAL EMOTIONAL REVERSAL (PER)

This third category is, like the second one, very common. Most people will have a brush with this one sooner or later. We may be completely congruent with being happy, healthy and successful, and congruent with our specific goals, yet still sabotage ourselves in less obvious ways than with specific or total reversal. And this self-sabotage can still ruin our lives, health and success. In PER we do not want to overcome all of the inconveniences we face; we want to keep some of them. For example, someone may have headaches on a daily basis, and when tested be congruent with 'I want to get rid of this headache,' but not congruent with 'I want to get rid of this headache completely.' This is a strange phenomenon that explains why a lot of people do not get completely well. They get better to a certain extent and hold on to the last vestige of their problem. What purpose can it possibly serve not to reach our goals completely, to keep some of our extra weight, disease, allergies, pain, cigarettes, cravings?

The main reason is that the subconscious mind would prefer that you get to your goal with the least effort possible. When you are sick and you become frustrated with being sick, you may want to be less sick and still get what you want. Let's take a situation where you learned as a young child that your mother was willing to take a day off work when you were sick and would give you all the pampering and attention you craved. Your subconscious mind becomes programmed to get you attention and pampering by making you sick. The only downside is that being sick in itself is not a whole lot of fun. So you get mostly better – but not completely better.

A high percentage of chronically ill people sabotage the last part of their recovery in this way. Let's look at a case history of a person with chronic fatigue syndrome.

CASE STUDY: PARTIAL EMOTIONAL REVERSAL

Paulina had seen, in her 12 years of being a chronic fatigue patient, over eight alternative doctors after exhausting every possibility in Western medical science, from Prozac to corticosteroid injections, to no avail. She furthermore had been treated by the best in alternative care, including treatments with acupuncture, homeopathy, chiropractic, herbal therapy, Qigong, yoga, meditation, flower essences and more. She would feel better for two to three months and get her hopes up, only to relapse shortly afterwards. It was driving her insane. One of the therapists was following a course at my academy for Omega Healing and had discussed her case with me. I agreed to meet her once and see if I could give the therapist any additional insights. He had done extensive testing on Paulina and had checked her for emotional reversal. She was a young woman in her thirties, good-looking and actually not looking ill at all. She told me that I was her last hope. I told her not to say that because sometimes we create diseases to allow us to find our spiritual path. When nothing of the external help we are seeking is working, we may turn inside to find out why we are manifesting this. I also told her that I could only be of support to her; her own body would do the rest.

Paulina was congruent with TER (Total Emotional Reversal), SER (Specific Emotional Reversal) *and* with PER. She remained strong on the statement:

'I want to completely get over this!'

And weak on:

'I do not want to keep any of this!'

Charly, her therapist and my student, had also tested her on this. So I followed my intuition and had her say the following:

'I want to keep just a tiny little bit of my chronic fatigue.'

She was again strong, indicating that this was true for her.

Charly was completely excited, as were Paulina and myself. We had the feeling that we had found her last little bit of resistance. I had learned something new and found out how important this was. We went on to try and discover her underlying reasons – not that they really matter, but just because it is fun to find out how the subconscious mind operates. As you will see later, knowing what incident caused the emotional blockage is not important; the only thing we really need to do is to let go of the past, whatever it held for us.

In Paulina's case, what emerged was that if the disease were to be completely healed, she would become responsible for taking care of the house, her two children and her part-time job as a graphic designer. Her subconscious mind did not think that was fair; she was the oldest of a family of four. Her family had always had financial problems. As the oldest sister, she was responsible for running the household and actually managing her two brothers and sister. Only when she was sick was she relieved from her duties. Her emotions were anger, disappointment, frustration and worry.

Paulina totally changed after this eight-minute session and was completely healed in the next six weeks. Normally, chronic fatigue conditions take more treatments, but in her case she had already been treated by reputable doctors and health practitioners; what we were working with was just the missing link.

In general, though, there is tremendous success with chronic fatigue cases and I would recommend anyone with such a condition to look into emotional balancing. It may change your life for the better, faster than with most therapies. What is important is that even if the subconscious mind wants a tiny little bit of disease, this will block complete healing. Sabotage is sabotage and can still ruin your life, relationships, marriages, exercising, losing weight, stop smoking and other areas of your life, such as finances and friendships.

Now let's look at the fourth and last category of reversal.

INCIDENTAL EMOTIONAL REVERSAL (IER)

This category could almost be called 'miscellaneous', because everything that does not fit in the first three categories can be considered IER. Falling into this category are a myriad of reasons why we subconsciously believe that we should not obtain our goals.

Timing

It may not be the right time for several reasons; maybe you just want to hold on to a problem – let's say in the case of an illness – until everyone is convinced it is a real disease and not an imaginary thing. So, if you suffer a little bit longer you can convince them. Maybe you'll have to wait until a certain person sees you the way you are and, once he or she has given you the attention or fulfilled your needs, you can let go. Maybe subconsciously you believe you should hold on to something harming you (or no longer helping you) because on some level you feel you haven't suffered enough; you need some more punishment. Maybe if you heal now, it would be bad timing because there is a big project coming up at work and you don't feel you should be asked to tackle it, because you are still weak. Maybe if you heal now you will get too many things coming at you at once.

Obviously the subconscious mind is very creative about coming up with reasons to keep you where you are. Of course, most reasons seem completely reasonable, and actually in most cases show prudence. But still it is all self-sabotage.

It Is Not Good for Others

This reason is used a lot. If we get well it may not be in the best interest of others. Maybe Mary is doing your job and, if you come back to work full-time now, it will create stress in the office. Your GP might be embarrassed that you were not cured by him; you have empathy for him after all he has done for you. Your spouse enjoys taking care of you and looking after everything; she feels great in that role and you would hate to interrupt that. The subconscious mind can come up with more reasons: it would be bad for your marriage, relationship, friendships and so forth.

It Is Not Good for You

There are many reasons why something you feel you want is not good for you. Having lots of money can be a nuisance and give you lots of headaches you are not prepared to deal with. It may be better to be just comfortable instead of shooting for the stars. Being responsible not only for your successes but also for your failures can also be a frightening prospect. You may have to forgive someone for what he has done to you, and don't actually feel prepared to do that. You may have the disempowering belief that you do not deserve success, that you are not worthy of it and thus you'd rather not have it. You may think you do not have all the skills you need to really make it all the way, or feel that maybe this objective requires someone with more courage and self-esteem than you currently have. Maybe you won't enjoy your success; maybe it is not really what you want; maybe you are overlooking something. Maybe it will cost you too much energy, time, money, your health, your relationship; it may inhibit your spiritual growth.

Again, we can only be in awe of how incredibly creative the subconscious mind is at making excuses. And do you know that it succeeds most of the time in tricking you into believing these roadblocks exist out there in reality? You become the marionette of your own mind and if you don't do something about it, you will be stuck in the same pattern over and over again.

The statements I use to uncover IER are diverse, but the easiest is: 'I do not want to have any reasons to sabotage myself.' Or we can ask the subconscious mind directly: 'Are there any other reasons for you still to sabotage your goal now or in the future? If you still have any reasons left, your muscles will test weak now!' If we get a weak muscle test, that would confirm that there are still some subconscious issues making you not totally congruent and continuing to sabotage yourself.

Any of these reversal categories can easily be treated. As we will see later, accepting that we *may* fail is key. By accepting this, we are accepting all our fears surrounding success, and can stop resisting what we want. It is a principle borrowed from martial arts: when you fight something, you struggle and lose lots of energy. You will win some and lose some. By completely relaxing and accepting defeat as a realistic possibility, we are more relaxed and less worried about the outcome and focus our energy where it matters.

CASE STUDY: INCIDENTAL EMOTIONAL REVERSAL

Sandra was 38 years old, a single mother with two boys: one nine years old, the other four. She was studying to become a naturopathic doctor and was juggling being a mum, studying and seeing some clients to make extra income. She was suffering with adhesive capsulitis – or, in simpler terms, 'frozen' shoulder. She could not pick up her four-year-old or comb her hair or perform certain movements, like reaching over her head to take something out of a kitchen cupboard. It was pretty annoying and several colleagues had tried in vain to help her with her shoulder. She was ready to get some steroid injections when her sister-in-law suggested she come see me. She had been treated extensively on an emotional level and that seemed to give her some temporarily relief, but after a short while she was back to square one.

Sandra tested fine for TER (Total Emotional Reversal), SER (Specific) and PER (Partial), but became weak for IER (Incidental) with the following statement: 'I want to completely let go of all the reasons for me having this shoulder condition.' This indicated an incongruence, so then I tested the reverse and she was strong (congruent) with it: 'I do not want to let go of all the reasons I have for having this shoulder condition.' She was also congruent with: 'It is not good for me to let go of this completely now!' 'It is not good for others if I let go of this completely now!' 'I do not want to enjoy my life without this shoulder condition!' and 'I do not deserve to be completely well!'

So, she had quite some issues left to work on. What came out was that her subconscious mind believed that she could not handle all she was handling, and that by doing all the things she was doing in her life, she did not have time to go out and meet men. By making her unable to do all of her chores, her subconscious mind was trying to create time for her to track down a suitable partner. Also, having a shoulder problem meant there were chores she could not do, like mowing the lawn or fixing the fence. Her subconscious mind hoped for a friendly unmarried neighbour to step in and that they would fall in love and live happily ever after. Getting better was also not good for her own mother, who loved to come and help out. Also, she felt she did not deserve to be completely well because her subconscious mind knew that she had so many defects and had committed so many mistakes in the past. So, for Sandra there were several reasons not to let go completely.

We worked for about 30 minutes to get all of the emotions blocking the energy channels to the shoulder resolved. After that she had full control over her shoulder and was completely healed. After 12 months she was still not in a relationship, but she was happy, had a new job and had moved to another city.

How do you feel now, knowing that you have a subconscious mind that will stop at nothing to get you what you want? So, you'd better be completely congruent with your goals and desires, and crystal clear on what you really want!

In Chapter 13 I will introduce some easy techniques I have developed to help you let go completely of any of the four reversal categories, and I will teach you an exercise to do every day, for just four to five minutes, that will eliminate these sabotage mechanisms for good.

I am happy to see you are still reading; that is an indication that you have got what it takes to be successful. Most people would already have been overruled by their subconscious mind to stop reading because if you follow through, your life may change dramatically. Be sure to read the next chapter which deals extensively with one of the most powerful and yet very simple healing techniques: *forgiveness.*

Time to Journal

What Are You Sabotaging?

Write down all the areas in life where you procrastinate, feel resistant to or self-sabotage, and start to practise becoming congruent by visualizing yourself actually committing to being successful in these areas. See how you are doing what you need to do in order to be successful. Keep practising every day until it feels natural for you to do whatever it takes to achieve your objectives.

CHAPTER 10

FORGIVENESS

Trudy looked at me, very upset. She came forward when I asked for a volunteer to do a demonstration of emotional balancing. She suffered from chronic hepatitis and fatigue. She was a school-teacher but had not worked for three years. What came out was that she had been sexually abused by three men, about five years previously. She suffered nightmares a couple of nights a week. The reason she was looking at me, upset, was that I'd told her that, in order to heal, she had to forgive those three men. She said, 'My hepatitis has nothing to do with those three men abusing me; this is too painful. I do not want to forgive them!' I told her that I understood how she felt and yet the fact that she did not forgive them was affecting her immune system and liver. I told her, 'You only have two options right now:

'**Option 1:** keep reliving the past over and over again and you will slowly but surely destroy yourself. Not only did they abuse you then. You *choose* to relive it; your bitterness will totally destroy you. Is it worth it?

'**Option 2:** you forgive them and release the past, heal and take your own life back. The choice is yours!'

Trudy finally understood what it was all about, and chose to forgive. We did an extensive forgiveness session. After that she started to cry, and you could see that this was the necessary outcome of holding on to those painful emotions for so long. Her chronic hepatitis completely cleared in the next eight weeks and she went back to work.

RELEASING THE PAST

In order to move forward and become the creators of our lives, we need to let go of the past and forgive everyone who we think has hurt us. We also need to forgive ourselves.

I have worked with forgiveness as part of my therapy for the last 20 years, with amazing results.

My rule about forgiveness is: *you can never forgive too much.*

Being unable or unwilling to forgive is the biggest silent killer in our Western civilized world. It can cause heart disease, cancer and weakening of the immune system; these three combined account for the majority of premature deaths. You want to become a Master in forgiving and learn how this can literally set you free from the past. The past is over and no longer changeable. What we can do is change how we feel and think about the past. We keep punishing ourselves in the present by not letting go of our resentments, guilt, criticism, hurt and fears from the past.

PARENTS AND FORGIVENESS

I strongly believe that we choose where, when and how we will incarnate. In my imagination I see the following happening before we reincarnate: we do a search to find the best parents, culture, country and genetics to serve our spiritual growth. When the perfect match has been found, we wait for our turn to incarnate. We even choose our date of birth to take advantage of the astrological forces that will have an effect on our lives. Maybe you think this is too far-fetched, but I do not believe so. I think we all choose *the perfect parents* for us to learn certain lessons which will enable us to grow spiritually. That is why some of us have chosen parents who fight all the time or are too busy to care for us or who are addicted to alcohol and cigarettes. This is all part of our karmic pattern, including also our gender, ethnic background, culture, family miasmas, country and religion. Our goal is to transcend all of that and discover that we cannot blame our parents for being who they are. We have chosen them exactly for those reasons. *They are perfect for what we want to accomplish.* We wanted them because they are imperfect and would treat us badly or not love us, abuse us or be any way they have been. For some reason we've needed all of this to achieve our spiritual goals. Sadly enough, we forget all of this and, when we are all grown up, we accuse them of not being perfect. We want to believe in fairy tales, and a part of us wants everything to be perfect, and that means that we really want no discomfort in any shape or form. That is impossible; if we want to grow and learn, we need to let go of the past and take control of the present moment. To do that, we need to look at our patterns, the situations we keep creating over and over. What are we looking for that we are not getting? The basic needs that we want from our parents, to feel loved, are:

1. **Acceptance**
2. **Understanding**
3. **Admiration**
4. **Acknowledgement**
5. **Recognition**
6. **Reassurance**
7. **Approval**
8. **Encouragement**
9. **Respect**
10. **Trust**
11. **Appreciation**
12. **Care**

When we do not get this from our parents, we will look elsewhere. It may be in sport (respect, admiration, acceptance, recognition, encouragement). It may be in school, in relationships, marriage, friendships or at work. Most of us will do a lot to get what we want or need – take some time to look at these 12 basic needs and seek the ones that resonate strongly with you. What do you do to get them?

I learned from a friend, Fiona Brouwer, a relationship counsellor who uses this in all of her sessions, to give what you need abundantly to others and to yourself. When you are in balance your needs will be negligible. And the first thing to do is to forgive our parents for all the misconceptions we've had about them. Our parents have been instrumental in how we are now, and the time has come to take over and create the image of ourselves that we really want.

A lot of parents blame their children for their problems or for not being there for them after all they have done for them. Don't buy into that crap and don't accept guilt, shame or any of that. Your parents have to develop spiritually as well, but it is their choice if they don't. You cannot carry their bitterness, resentment, guilt and fear for them; they have to learn to be at peace with themselves. Send them love and help where you can, and let go of any negative feelings imposed on you!

HEALING THE HEART

Many of us have been hurt by others. Your spouse has left you for another, your mother was too busy to care for you, your father was very strict and told you many times you are worthless. Some people have experienced rape, incest or violence. There are many ways to be hurt. A loved one killed by a drunk driver or shot by a thief can seem a particularly senseless tragedy. Such events can fill us with bitterness, resentment and feelings of hatred or revenge. You keep on thinking *Why?* You cannot accept the idea that this has happened. Forgiveness is the solution to healing the heart, finding inner peace and letting go of all emotional wounds. For many people it is not easy to forgive; the concept is alien to them. They want justice, and see forgiveness as letting the other person off the hook. You will understand by now that by not forgiving you are trapping yourself in a never-ending past, losing tremendous quantities of life-force in the process.

Over the years I have been asked many questions about forgiveness:

- What do I do if I don't feel it is right to forgive?
- Do I need to tell the person that I forgive him?
- Do I forgive her even if she doesn't care and did not show remorse?
- How do I forgive God?

- If I have created all this myself, why should I forgive someone else who was part of my creation?
- Do I need to make up with the people I forgive?
- How do I let go of the thoughts of revenge and pain?
- What if I forgive and they abuse me again?
- What if the person does not stop trying to insult me and hurt me?

These and more questions are asked over and over again, and they are not always easy to answer. The idea of forgiving someone who has hurt you can be very controversial and at times confusing, so let's take a look at what forgiveness really is and why we fight it so much. We will also look at the energetic blocks we cause by not forgiving. We will discuss forgiving yourself, God and others. After you forgive, the healing can start; we will also look at how you can speed up this healing with the 14 gateways. We will discuss the difference between mental forgiveness and forgiveness from the bottom of your heart.

WE ARE ALL ONE

First of all we need to understand that we are part of a whole, and that nothing happens independently of that whole. What happens to each of us is part of our collective consciousness. We create our own reality – every second of it. This is the first concept we need to accept in order to understand why certain things happen to us. The term 'collective consciousness' comes from the sociologist Emile Durkheim; Edgar Cayce introduced us to the notion of Akashic records, and Rupert Sheldrake talks about the morphogenetic field. We, all of us, influence and form these collective fields by our thoughts, actions – and our ability to forgive. By our acts of compassion and our willingness to transcend our own creations, we shape this consciousness. The resonating effect of many small acts of love and compassion fortifies the forces that transform the world. We are an integral part of changing the world's consciousness by our deeds, thoughts and feelings. We have the karmic choice to feed the collective consciousness with the energy of resentment, fear, bitterness, frustration and so on, or with the healing energy of love, forgiveness, joy and compassion. The choice is really yours: either you will choose to create a better world or to continue the negative energies that caused you pain in the first place. In short, it does not matter if your intention is to transform yourself or the world; the two are intertwined. This power is ours; everybody has it, no exceptions. The question is whether you are ready, willing and able to take responsibility for playing your part or if you will cling to the idea, 'What does it matter what I do? I am just one person.' So, rather than feed that disempowering thought, focus on the process of transforming yourself and, in doing that, help to change the world with your intention and consciousness.

The first step is to look more closely at the concept of forgiveness.

CASE STUDY

Hal was a Vietnam veteran and he was also an alcoholic. He had inherited quite a fortune and could permit himself all the luxury he wanted. The thing he wanted most was inner peace. This case study took place when I was on holiday in Hawaii and having a good time. I was muscle-testing a man in his early forties because he wanted to lose weight. As we were working, Hal passed by and asked, 'What are you guys doing?' It was indeed kind of strange to see two grown-ups playing with each other's hands on the beach. I explained to him the concept of muscle-testing and how I was making this other fellow congruent with letting go of his cravings for chocolate. Hal got interested and asked me if I had ever worked with war veterans. I said yes, and that in general the results were very good. He asked me to test him and I agreed to see him later. After half an hour we met and he told me his story. The thing that he could not let go of was an incident in which he came eye to eye with a Vietcong officer. Both pulled their guns simultaneously. Hal's shot got the other man in the chest and the Vietcong officer's shot missed him. Every night this event happened over and over again in his dreams. He could not get rid of the look in the eyes of his opponent as he was shot in the heart and died.

I tested Hal and the only emotion that came up was that he was unforgiving toward himself. We did a forgiveness session together and he forgave himself for taking a life to save his own. Hal cried silently for 10 minutes and felt a tremendous relief. After that session Hal had no more nightmares and stopped drinking, cold turkey. I helped him in rehab and with the physical symptoms that go with that, and two days later he was completely changed. This is another example of the healing power of forgiveness.

COMING OUT OF DENIAL

In order to forgive, it is important that we be completely honest with ourselves. If we are in denial, forgiveness will not work. Thoughts are the emotions translated into incentives to act. Thoughts lead to actions, choices, decisions. Emotional honesty is about taking your responsibility and not hiding behind excuses. You cannot truly forgive if you have not faced events fully. If you fail to acknowledge your feelings, you are failing to forgive. We have to come to terms with how deeply we have been hurt. We need to understand that only by our ability to love can we heal ourselves, and *especially* when a painful event makes no sense to us whatsoever. If you accept that the goal of this journey we call life is our spiritual evolution, why shouldn't we forgive? By not forgiving you are hurting only yourself. Maybe you have even created situations so you can take a big step toward your spiritual awareness.

We also need to face the emotions that will stop us from forgiving, that keep us shackled to the past and are the cause of many of our ailments. The mind will give us plenty of reasons to stay unforgiving. We want revenge and justice; we keep holding on to our bitterness as a warning to keep our focus on preventing something similar ever happening again. Sometimes we want time for the pain to lessen and then it will be easier to forgive. Do not be fooled by this one. It can take years and years before we even come close to forgiveness, especially when we have experienced rape, incest or the death of a loved one. We are giving our health away by waiting for forgiveness; when you get a cancer diagnosis or have a heart attack it is too late, the damage is done.

Forgiveness should not be a 'comfortable' act; it can be very painful. It is about coming out of denial. We deny the fact that we are the only one who is damaged by holding on to the past. We deny the fact that we need to forgive in order to get on with our lives. Embracing forgiveness is the best thing you can ever do for yourself.

THE CONSEQUENCES OF FORGIVENESS

Resentment, hostility, anger, revenge, bitterness, frustration and being unforgiving are very detrimental to our health. They primarily affect the liver and, secondarily, the heart and thymus (immune system). By holding on to these emotions we slowly but surely undermine our health and mental state. Precious life-force is lost. By forgiving we assume responsibility and let go of wanting revenge. What we are doing is letting go on the physical and energetic plane, and giving our pain to the highest source. Only by letting go can we be healed emotionally.

We need to differentiate, however, between forgiveness from the mind and forgiveness from the heart. Forgiveness from the mind is when we understand on an intellectual level that it is better to forgive. It is the right thing to do. So we 'forgive' by suppressing our true feelings. This is even worse than not forgiving, because we may be led to believe that we have forgiven, while in reality we have not. I have encountered this many times. This is in the same category as denial. Heartfelt forgiveness is when we accept our responsibility for creating our own hurt, and we accept that the other person was just a part of it. We can actually thank him or her for the lesson and wish the other person well by connecting to the universal love we have deep in our hearts. We must still deal with the emotions that may arise, especially if we meet this person again; we may feel pain and all kinds of emotions, which will feel even worse if he or she doesn't show remorse.

Remember: forgiveness is not about the other person; it is only about you!

There are many misconceptions about forgiveness. Some people think they have to *tell* the person who has offended them that they have been forgiven; this is not necessary. You can forgive and never raise the issue, unless you think you can influence an ongoing behaviour and offer some insights that may help the other person change. But that is only if you feel up to it (see page 210 for advice on how to do this effectively, without being confrontational).

Other people say that by forgiving someone you are acknowledging that you were in the wrong. This is not the case. By forgiving someone we are releasing negative energy. Forgiving someone does not mean that you feel the destructive behaviour was OK, or that the person did not know what she was doing. And you don't have to forget what happened; we are here to learn our lessons and thus become better at creating what serves us. Once the emotional charge is gone from the incident, we can let go of it while keeping hold of the insights. Forgiveness does not mean we have to go back and pretend nothing happened. We don't have to stay in a dysfunctional relationship, nor do we have to try and restore a broken one. Reconciliation may be a possibility but only if it feels right for you.

Some people believe they should blame instead of forgiving. Blaming your parents will only destroy you, and you will not profit from the healing that comes from releasing your emotional bondage. Your parents had only one duty, and that was to look after you until you were old enough to look after yourself. Once you were able to take care of yourself, their duty was finished and your spiritual journey began. The first step is realizing that they were exactly as you wanted them to be; now you can support their growth by loving them as they are without any blaming or finger-pointing.

You can choose how you feel about the past and change its meaning. How would you feel if your children blamed you for everything that did not work in their lives? Blaming has not helped anyone yet. Blaming is another way to stay stuck in the past.

Forgiveness is not easy; anyone who says it is easy may be a master of intellectual forgiveness, but forgiving from the heart entails much more. Forgiveness is a decision and does not require a process; it should be instantaneous and from the heart, because we understand the workings of the universe. The sooner we focus on forgiving, the easier it becomes to do. By forgiving we immediately go along the path to emotional healing. We do not need to know all the facts in order to be able to forgive – they are not important. The only thing that is important is our willingness to forgive and release the emotional chains to the past. It is like releasing a hostage: you!

UNFINISHED BUSINESS

Not having forgiven is unfinished business that has an effect on your energy fields. It creates a disharmonic resonance that may lead to attracting more of the same. Chronic grief often comes out of feelings of loss, of not being able to let go of something we should let go of. Our intention with forgiveness is to finish something we have not finished without disregarding our own self. We need patience to finish the process of emotional healing. Forgiveness is a choice, and choice is karma. By forgiving we are also releasing negative karma. We let go of bitterness, grief, frustration, anger and other harmful emotions. Therefore forgiveness causes inner calm and peace. Forgiveness has nothing to do with justice or getting satisfaction because the offender is punished. Forgiveness is an act of mercy and trust in the laws of the universe. It is not for us to judge and punish. We actually relinquish our rights for the pain we suffered. That is why it is so difficult. Forgiveness starts with you being willing to take that decision to release the offender from what he or she has done to you. Forgiveness is releasing your hostages and prisoners, finishing the unfinished business, cleaning up your energy field and breaking karmic chains from the past.

WHOM TO FORGIVE

We live in a society where many people are out only to satisfy their own needs. They even take what is not theirs and may inflict a lot of pain in that process. Sometimes they have the conscious intention to cause others pain or harm, whereas sometimes you are an innocent bystander who got caught in the crossfire. Others are not always aware of what they are doing and how their actions affect other people. Some are repeat offenders and will go on with their destructive behaviour until they are caught. Many you may never see again; some you may have to face on a regular basis. Some will repent and ask for forgiveness, while most won't. Does this make it any easier? The answer is: it does not matter at all. It is not for you to change their lives; you have to deal with one person and that's you. We could forgive them all – those we know and those we don't know. We could forgive the ones who did something horrible and the ones who hurt our feelings by making negative remarks. We could forgive those who show remorse and those who don't. The truth is that every second we live without finishing this process, we are hurting ourselves. How long do you want to wait?

Even if someone keeps offending you, you have to forgive them. Also, you can work on yourself until their actions no longer affect you emotionally.

If you want to become good at healing yourself, you have to learn to forgive immediately. Every day many things happen at which we can take offence; as soon as you notice that, learn to forgive and let go. The better you get at this, the less you'll end up with unfinished business and the less toxic build-up you'll create. Do not avoid the offender; this person is there to teach you about inner peace, love and forgiveness until you can feel good no matter what he says. You are now ready to move on. No offence is too big to be forgiven. And the offence is not even the issue when we are forgiving. The bigger the pain, the more motivated we should be to let go. Even those events that are so devastating that they seem almost impossible to forgive should be forgiven.

Just remember: *you cannot forgive too much; you cannot forgive enough!*

It does not matter how many times we have been insulted, offended, humiliated or abused; we must forgive even the worst of the worst to be set free. This is the essence of healing. It is never easy or uncomplicated, but we have a choice and by choosing forgiveness we are utilizing the Source of love within us that resembles the grace and mercy of God. Each time we forgive we are climbing another rung on our ladder of spiritual evolution. When we become good at this, fewer things will hurt us because we will start understanding the workings of the reality we help to create.

HOW TO FORGIVE

Many people ask how to forgive, how actually to execute their decision to forgive. This is in truth the easiest part, and there are no set rules for how to do it. I will discuss here how I coach people to do it and what else we can do to let the healing take place.

The first thing is that forgiveness can be done anywhere; you don't need to go to any special place or confront anyone. It is something you do in the privacy of your own home. Some people you will forgive may already have died, others you may not even know the names of. Even if the person is available, you don't have to go to her and say, 'I have forgiven you!' Some offenders may not even be aware that they have hurt you. It is not your task to judge them; leave that up to God and the laws of the universe. That does not mean that if a person's behaviour is a source of irritation, you cannot confront him in a loving way and ask him to change it. But once you do, it is up to the person whether to change or not; your job is done.

Forgiveness is a spiritual act which brings you closer to God (whatever God is for you) and will start the healing process immediately. It is between you and your highest consciousness, which is part of all, which is God. The only eyewitness you will need is God. There is no need to tell anyone, especially not if you don't want to show off your goodness. If the subject comes up, you can always talk about it. You can talk to someone when you are in the healing process that takes place after you have forgiven. More important is to forgive and leave the details to the universe. You are done; you are clean. You have restored your power and have tapped into your unconditional love.

For me, God is the personification of grace. The philosophy of reincarnation is appealing because it is a confirmation of God's love, mercy and fairness. It helps us to understand that every incident has its purpose; children starving in Bangladesh, deaths due to accidents, wars, cancer and other preventable diseases. God is not to blame; we create all of this and, because of our free choice, we get what we create. Due to the laws of karma, the philosophy of reincarnation becomes the force of justice that cannot be bent. By creating harmony in our lives and those around us, we are harmonizing with unconditional love. By choosing to forgive we are also choosing grace. We allow more magic into our hearts.

FORGIVENESS SESSION

When you forgive it is always good to connect to the Source of unconditional love, to feel God's love for all creation, and then be able to release the pain in that loving moment. So, the best thing to do is to find a quiet place where you have privacy and can take a moment for yourself without being interrupted. You can sit in your car, your bedroom, take a walk or find a quiet place. Then, what I normally recommend is to sit comfortably or to lie on your back and put both hands on your heart. Breathe in and out slowly and relax completely. Focus on your heart and connect your heart with the unconditional love around you; feel the energy of love go through your body. Think about all the things written in this and the previous chapter: that we choose our parents to assist our growth and that we are creating, moment by moment, our lives. This painful incident, too, has been created for us to confront. What lessons have you learned? Maybe it is just the fact that you should forgive even if every cell in your body does not think it is fair. Send your love to the person who hurt you and forgive him or her. Also come to terms with the fact that you will not seek revenge or fight back, but use that energy to heal your heart instead. Then, in your mind, destroy the record of wrongs done to you and add to your list of lessons learned.

With emotional balancing we proceed to the next step and now work on the energy of the meridians in our body. First, treat the liver energy; this is where our anger, resentment, frustration and guilt are locked away. Massage or treat this point while saying, 'I deeply love and accept myself with my anger [or resentment, or feelings of revenge] toward [the offender].' Repeat this at least three times or until you feel calm and peaceful and it is not stressful to visualize or think of this person (the liver point is on the right side, halfway up the arc of your ribcage). Then you move to the kidney points (located next to the breastbone, under the clavicles), which deal with fear. If we do not deal with our fears, we may project the incident and recreate something similar in future. While massaging the two kidney points, say, 'I deeply love and accept myself with my fears that something like this might happen again!' Again, repeat this at least three times or until you feel totally comfortable and peaceful inside. Then, for the last part of this forgiveness session, massage the points of the heart, next to the cuticle on the inside of both little fingers. Massage or treat these alternately, again a minimum of three or so times until you feel completely peaceful. The affirmation is: 'I deeply love and forgive myself for creating this incident and I forgive [the offender] for being part of this and I let go of this, now and forever!'

That is the whole forgiveness session: we deal with our anger/resentment, our fears of this happening again, and then we forgive ourselves and the offender for what has occurred. If you have also felt angry toward God, you can add the following affirmation (while treating the heart points): 'I deeply love and forgive myself for blaming God for this incident; please forgive me, God, for my ignorance!'

This forgiveness session has helped thousands of people to initiate their healing, and I have seen many chronic diseases get much better or heal completely once a person is ready, able and willing to let go of the past.

So... are you ready? Is there anyone you want to forgive now? Including yourself? You can start now; make a list of all the people or incidents that have caused you pain. There is no better time than now!

SOME LAST ARGUMENTS IN FAVOUR OF FORGIVENESS

So, you have done the only right thing, confronted yourself and have forgiven everyone who needed to be forgiven, including yourself. It should be over and you can get on with your life, right?

In many instances this will be an illusion. Your decision and act of forgiveness may be attacked, ridiculed by others. Your subconscious mind may also protest and create doubt in you. Your thoughts may not be in line with your deed and you may feel bad about it. This is normal; *after forgiveness the real healing starts* – and it may not be a smooth ride. So, be prepared for the face-off. If you have not forgiven your own mistakes and failures, you keep a space open for self-condemnation. Many people carry guilt around with them; guilt because their children have not turned out to be exemplary citizens, guilt due to divorce, guilt because they've been involved in a car accident that injured others badly, guilt because they were a bad example to their children, guilt because they've made many mistakes. There are so many reasons to feel guilty! Maybe you blame yourself for a broken marriage or a lost loved one. Some of these things may have genuinely been your fault: if you had paid a little bit more attention, if you hadn't had that drink, or fallen asleep and so on. Please make a list of the things you blame yourself for, because these should be addressed as soon as possible.

Many of us feel inadequate because we cannot live up to our own expectations. We have given up on our dreams and have accepted our limitations. But we still blame ourselves. Our self-image is completely distorted and not close to reality. We try to fit in and the ongoing barrage of beautiful bodies on TV and in advertisements does not help much. We buy into those illusions and try to keep up with a battle that most of us will lose. Take a moment now and do a forgiveness session on yourself and become more comfortable with who you are, the good and the bad. Accept and love yourself deeply; you deserve it and you've earned peace of mind.

Some of you may still not be open to forgiving someone because you feel what happened was beyond all reason. You feel it was just too much, too cold-blooded, too calculated – this person deserves to be punished and put away for good! If you choose to hold on to the incident, you are choosing to relive it over and over again. In other words: there is a part of you that must be masochistic and enjoys pain. That is the only reason for you to hold on at this point, knowing that through forgiveness you would heal yourself, knowing that forgiveness does not say anything about the other, but everything about you. You choose to continue on the path of pain and self-destruction. Fair enough; everyone has the right to make his own choices. But know this: you choose spiritual darkness instead of spiritual enlightenment when you choose not to forgive. No matter how painful, we can always forgive. Millions have forgiven the worst offences, and so can you!

LET THE HEALING START

After forgiveness we embark on the path of healing and harmony. We may still be shaken, but we are determined to heal ourselves and put all this behind us. Once in a while we will have to struggle to maintain our choice of forgiveness, but that is the only way to tap into the healing energy of love. By not forgiving we constrict our hearts and diminish our connection with our deepest spiritual level.

You may need some time for the healing to complete its course; until then it is best to keep on working on the negative painful emotions. Visualize yourself meeting the offender and feel completely calm and loving. With the techniques in Part II, you can eliminate any remaining pain. It is important not to try to avoid confrontation at all costs; that may be a form of denial. Keep your focus on your objective to let go of all the past pain. Also, do not retaliate by ignoring the other person or treating him or her harshly. See it as part of your healing journey and a way to test yourself to check if the healing is complete. It is normal to experience inner turbulence. That is your compass. Expect to have some painful moments, and take time to think about how you will deal with them in advance.

Time to Journal
Whom Do You Need to Forgive?

Start today with forgiving at least three people a day until you have cleared your list completely. After each forgiveness session, visualize this person and check how you feel. If you still feel some emotion or resentment, you are not done.

Repeat this process for seven days in a row until you feel neutral or comfortable when thinking about this person or situation.

Forgiveness is only done completely if you can wish for them what you wish for yourself: that they may find peace and happiness in their lives.

YOUR THOUGHTS CAN BE CHANGED

No matter how severe or cruel the incident was, the meaning we give it is the consequence of our inner thoughts and our past experiences. Your thinking creates the feelings and you accept those feelings as true and real. If you change your thoughts, the feelings will change as well.

Remember, the past only has power over you if you give it that power. If you choose again to live in the now, you release yourself from the past. We can start all over without the pain or stress. We choose even our thoughts, and we can choose to have other thoughts. That is the incredible power bestowed upon us. You can be strong and reject all thoughts that sap your life-force; you don't have to settle. Let go of self-hatred, resentment, guilt and blame; these are very negative. By focusing on the thought as it occurs, we can prevent ourselves from ending up in a negative self-defeating spiral.

By changing your thoughts, you tap into the powerful healing energy we all have in our bodies and can feel loving energy flowing through you. Every thought in your mind should be checked to see if it fits into your new pattern and spiritual path. Observe how you think and judge, and alter negative thoughts immediately. Do not expect instant change, however; be prepared for battle and, by keeping your attention on balancing your emotions, you will triumph sooner than you think.

CONFRONTATION

It is sometimes good to share your pain with others as long as you do not get into 'victim mode'. By choosing to be a victim you block your growth and your healing. This is what Carolyne Myss calls *woundology*: using our emotional wounds to get attention and care from others. This will keep you captive. It is best to maintain a non-judgemental attitude toward your offender, an attitude of understanding and a willingness to see the pain that has led to his or her behaviour. Place value on the people who hurt you, find something in them that is positive and see them as people struggling on their own spiritual path. Refuse to fight and find love in your heart. It is a good idea to pray for them and send them love every day; this can help to transform the world. Every prayer goes to the collective consciousness and helps to promote global healing. When you do this you will notice that your emotional pain begins to diminish and, sooner or later, it will be completely gone. Then you can ask yourself if it is necessary to confront your offender. It is only worthwhile if you can operate from a place of love and inner peace. It can also be useful if this can lead to a change of the offensive behaviour. Speak the truth in love without placing blame, and explain exactly what is offensive in the other person's behaviour. Your motives must be pure otherwise you are just fooling yourself and are actually seeking some sort of vengeance.

If possible, check with others if they have had the same experience, but do not hide behind them; speak only for yourself. In some cases, if innocent lives are in danger, you may seek to contact the appropriate authorities to deal with the situation.

Sometimes it is wiser not to confront someone if you know it is useless or may even make matters worse. Sometimes it is not up to you to do the confronting, and at other times you may not have all the facts. Think before the confrontation about the best way to go about this. You have to be ready, your wounds healed, your heart at peace. Sometimes it is best to ask the other person for forgiveness first, say for something that he or she might have taken as offensive. In this way you open the door more easily for the other person to address his or her own behaviour. You must also be willing to open your heart and show the other you really care and you are not out for revenge. Being sensitive to his or her circumstances and pain makes this easier. Also, think of safety first: if the offender has a quick temper and an inclination toward violence, you may prefer to speak to him or her at a distance, by ringing, writing a letter or email, or meeting up in a public place. You don't want to endanger yourself. Sometimes it is not practical to meet the person, due to distance or because it may just be too painful.

If you choose to write a letter, make sure to give it some careful thought. You may need to rewrite it a few times to find the best approach. Write from love, not from your pain. Read the letter back a few times: does it express your love, and have you also asked for forgiveness for the mistakes you made yourself? Remember to focus on love and the positive lessons you have learned from all of this.

SPIRITUAL PATH

The whole purpose of forgiveness is to initiate your own healing process, to allow you to get back to your spiritual path. Forgiveness is one of the spiritual exercises that can demand a lot from us. We need to practise until we become good at it. The better at it you become, the more you will notice that no one can really hurt you. You can *allow* someone to hurt you, but that is up to you. Your spirit is untouchable. Your body can be abused, but your spirit can rise above all. Once this is clear, it is easy to forgive. You will also start noticing how many people are unaware of the pain they inflict on others. You will see other people who are in severe pain themselves and want to hurt others because it is not fair that they have all this pain. So, you will start seeing people in a way you have not seen them before. People will try to hurt you because they feel that you have hurt them. It may be something simple like not giving them attention. It may be jealousy; maybe you spend more time with someone else. I have seen it all. People behave impulsively without thinking, even the people you expect to be more in tune, because they are 'spiritual'. The best attitude is not to expect anything, so you cannot be disappointed. Accept everyone just as they are, with all the good but also the bad. Do not try to change anyone, except yourself. Become a master of forgiveness, because then you tap into the universal love.

Time to Journal

With Whom Do You Have Unfinished Business?

Write down the names of people with whom you have unfinished business, and also write down the steps you will take to resolve this unfinished karma and a date when you will take the necessary actions. Check this list weekly until all is done.

CHAPTER 11

THE PARADOX OF AWARENESS

TO LEARN OR NOT TO LEARN

Many people believe we are here to learn lessons and grow spiritually. The truth is that we have nothing to learn whatsoever. We don't have to do anything to become a better or more spiritual person. We are already the best we can be. The only choice is whether or not to become *conscious* about it. If we choose, we can wake up to ourselves and experience the ultimate experience, the most celestial and godly experience of all: to remember and reconnect with who we really are.

The following story illustrates this.

The Eagle That Thought It Was a Chicken

A farmer's boy was hiking up in the mountains and discovered an eagle's nest with an egg in it. He took the egg back with him to the farm and put it in with the chicken eggs. When the eagle hatched, it thought it was a chicken. The eagle grew up and behaved like a chicken, eating worms and insects and clucking. Just like the other chickens, it would fly only a few feet into the air. The eagle lived all its life as a chicken, and grew to a very old age. One day it looked up and saw a beautiful bird circling above the farm. This bird was using the wind to glide along gracefully. The eagle was in complete awe of such magnificence. 'What kind of bird is that?' it asked. A nearby chicken answered, 'That is the king of all birds: an eagle. An eagle belongs to the sky like chickens belong to the earth.' The eagle died as a chicken because that was its perception of what it was.

Are You an Eagle or a Chicken? Or an Eagle Who Believes He's a Chicken?

If we don't become aware of our magnificence, we will always behave like the eagle who believed it was a chicken. Actually, most people prefer to be chickens; the reason is that, for most, that is comfortable. Waking up from this illusion is not pleasurable. It means we have to give up many of our limiting beliefs. It means that we have to act and be *as we truly are.*

The sad truth is that most people don't really want to become aware and experience their magnificence. The first step we need to make is to realize we are in denial and to become honest with ourselves. We have been in denial for so long that what we have appears real; we start to believe our own illusions. We have learned to be happy in relation to what we have, not what we are. When we don't have what we want, we are unhappy and we deny our eternal being, who is unconditionally happy. We don't want to give up getting something for our efforts. We want to see our desires met. The biggest challenge to becoming aware is being willing to open up to a new realm, to let go of the past.

Are you ready to let go of all your old beliefs? How much of the truth can you handle? Most of us are afraid of letting go of what we know, of living on the edge of the unknown, of exchanging our illusions for reality.

WHEN THERE IS NO PAST OR FUTURE, WHAT REMAINS IS A 'PRESENT'

The reality is: there is no past and there is no future. There is only now. The past is gone and the future is a mystery. Your now is a present that you give yourself. Can you see the beauty in the now? Can you be grateful for all that you are, and what you have created? Can you stop judging what is good or what would be best and just indulge in the experience that your soul is having right now? Can you heal whatever needs to be healed? Enjoy what there is to enjoy, and speak of what wants to be spoken through you?

Ponder these questions, because then you will grasp who you are and why you are here: to have an experience, to be in the experience. Don't worry about meaning; meaning will come later when the experience ends and becomes the experiment that you came to know in this dimension.

THE NOW ENCOMPASSES EVERYTHING: PAST, PRESENT AND WHAT IS TO BE

Actually the past and the future are right now. Many people strive after what they don't have. What about focusing on what you have created now, so you understand how you created it? By becoming an observer without judgement we can transform ourselves. To become enlightened means to become aware. First you observe what is happening in your life; you realize that you have created these scenarios yourself. So, in order to create a certain situation, you had to think certain thoughts – and once you realize this, you move on to the awareness of your thoughts. Then you realize that someone is having these thoughts, and that someone is you.

The spiritual masters tell us that the prime question in life is: 'Who am I? What is this entity I call "I"?' We can understand everything about computers, how to cook food, how to do many things, but if we do not know who the 'I' is, we are still unconscious, not knowing what is really going on in the world.

AWAKENING

The first step to rouse yourself from unconsciousness is to realize that you want to wake up. Do you understand this? The question is: who is doing the understanding of this? To look at the 'I' and become an observer; this will make you discover that you are not free, you are a slave of past conditioning, beliefs that do not serve you, fears you borrowed from your parents, family and teachers. You have become a product of your past experiences and programming.

Free will is a farce if you do not wake up. You are stuck in patterns of what you believe is right or wrong. You are so stuck that you cannot see that everyone else is stuck as well. Everybody is defending their own turf. We make our lives a misery and, like everyone else, believe that it's other people who make us miserable! The truth is that nobody can *make* you miserable if you are truly awake.

MEET THE GENIUS WHO CREATED THE PLAN FOR YOUR LIFE

There is no one to blame for anything; everything is going according to 'the plan'. Who made this Divine plan? You did! You are the genius behind this plan; there is no one else to blame, and you've been clever at creating a plan that has challenged you since the time you arrived in the dream state we call life. Congratulations, you are smarter than Einstein. Now you only have to remember: what was the plan?

Many people ask me, 'Why are we here?' My answer is the biggest paradox of all: 'We are here to find out why we are here!' Our goal is to remember our purpose, to analyze what has happened and find ways to discover who we really are.

It is painful to realize we have got sidetracked and now believe that certain things are true which are not. It is painful to emerge from unconsciousness and realize that you have been living an illusion.

WHO IS READING THIS BOOK?

Who is the person reading this sentence? Who is the reader? Who is the thinker? Who is the observer? Can the observer get to know himself? To understand and define the 'I', we need to know first what it is *not*. God (or whatever you call the spiritual source) is the biggest observer of all. God is the 'I' of all there is, all there was and all there ever will be. My 'I' is part of the godly 'I'. 'I' am a part of the total universal manifestation. God is universal love, so 'I' must be part of universal love.

What am 'I' not? 'I' am not my thoughts. Although I may have many thoughts – according to some scientists 60,000 of them a day – I am not my thoughts. I do recycle many of my thoughts, up to 90 per cent or more. I keep thinking, but I am not my thoughts.

'I AM SO I AM!'

I asked myself the question, 'Am I somebody?' The reality is that I use this body to experience certain sensations (feelings) that I can only experience when I lower my vibrational speed. The body is my 'spacesuit', created to explore slower vibrational energy. I slow myself down and limit myself by confining myself to this body. Another paradox is that birth (putting on this spacesuit) was a serious limitation of my being. By becoming human, 'I' died to be born. Life is a limited experience. Why would I want that? In one of my workshops, participants walk around for a day blindfolded. For most people this is a very scary experience. They need to rely on others and their other senses. Almost everyone discovers new things about themselves that can change their lives. They discover things they would not have discovered if they were not limited by the loss of sight. The same thing happens when the 'I' limits itself by incarnating. It will discover new aspects of itself that are almost impossible to know when there are no limitations.

So, 'I' am not my body. I am an entity that inhabits and controls this body. Our bodies change constantly; the only constant is the 'I'.

I am not my beliefs; beliefs can change. I am not my work. Some people say: 'I am a lawyer/doctor/clerk.' That is not true; you cannot just be a lawyer, doctor or clerk. Actually, these are limitations of who you are. A great deal of people box themselves in and become their own limitations. We create labels for our limitations, and then identify with those labels. Same with emotions: 'I am angry, I am sad.' That is a faulty use of language; the correct way to say this is, 'I feel this sensation inside of me that I have labelled anger (or sadness, or fear).' The 'I' is none of these boxes or labels. The 'I' is infinitely bigger than that. I-dentification with labels is what creates suffering and pain. The 'I' cannot suffer. When you step out of the suffering you observe that it's not the 'I' that is suffering. 'I' is I-nfinite, I-mmortal and is not I-dentifying with our earthly desires, labels, wants and needs. It's these desires, wants and needs that are the illusion we buy into and feel that we need to feel 'well'.

SUFFERING IS ATTACHMENT TO DESIRES AND EXPECTATIONS

All suffering eventually comes from desire. Desire comes from our memory (karma); it is only when we believe that we need things that we feel unfulfilled and get out of the state of 'being' and into acting to get what we desire.

Most people believe that if they can have *what they do not have, they will* be *more happy, secure, loved or peaceful.* So they start taking 'action' to get what they want, and in the meantime they are not 'being'. Many people have spent their lives pursuing what they don't have, and never being what they truly want to be. Just look around you: are most of the people you know doing things to get what they don't have so they can achieve some kind of desired state? What about you? Here is how it is for most of us: *Desire* → *Action* → *Desired state.*

The paradox is that we can be any way we want, once we understand that it is a choice.

If you want to be happy, start being happy right now; let go of your misery and suffering and immediately choose to be happy, no matter what. When you are in this state and are doing things from this attitude, you will attract more things that make you happy and you will have all you desire.

CHOOSE HAPPINESS

When we awaken from unconsciousness, we will realize that everything that has happened in our lives has been perfect for us. We have conspired with thousands, maybe millions if not billions, of other souls to create exactly the perfect circumstances to get where we are now and to read this book. One of the biggest breakthroughs in my life was when I quit worrying about what other people thought of me. I was really free to do what I felt best for me. You become free only when you stop needing approval from external sources. So, to reach the third level of happiness we need to realize that *happiness is a choice, not a result or outcome.* The key to getting all you want is to start feeling like you already have what you want.

Shape Your Inner World Until You Become It

In other words: start living the fantasy first with all your senses: visualize it, allow the feeling as if it were as real as real can get, feel the sensation of being and having every day, so your brain will be inundated with pleasure hormones and will form the synapses that create a magnetic force to attract what you dream of with grace, ease and joy.

By deciding how to feel, you create the conditions that are best for you. The process of creation starts with engaging all your senses and feeling it in your body; you then create a radiance that will set in motion the cosmic laws of manifestation that will attract what you want. This is always true.

So, here comes the next paradox: *if you do not get what you want or if you get what you* don't *want, it must mean that a part of you wants what you have got.* In other words: your conscious and unconscious are not congruent. By uniting the body, mind and spirit in experiencing in advance what you want in full colour, full of feeling and full of detail, you are literally shaping it and becoming it (it's your virtual reality).

When you add some 'spiritual spice' to this recipe, you are creating magic. The 'spiritual spice' is: *giving others what you desire most*, or *helping others get what they want*. The other spiritual ingredient is to do it from your heart, so that you genuinely want others to be as happy as you. The last and most important ingredient is that, once you shape this in your mind, you can enjoy it without becoming attached to it. What you already are, you are creating effortlessly. By being it, you can shape it and manifest it, easily and without effort. The universe becomes your helper. It will help you to get more of what you already have. So, if you are experiencing misery – that will lead to more misery. By helping others, by giving them what you have in abundance, more will come to you. You will become a magnet for what you are experiencing. Everything in your life so far was created and attracted by you; you have shaped it. All of it has had a purpose; it was part of your beliefs, healing or experiences.

If you want to change what you feel, start with feeling what you want and you will shape your destiny accordingly. Here is your choice now: do you want to create consciously or unconsciously? Creating unconsciously means letting your old programming take over; wouldn't you rather be the conscious creator of your destiny? You can be unconscious or you can be fully awake. The choice is yours. Are you one of the many or apart from the many? If you realize that everything is interconnected, and you understand that what you give to others is the same as what you give to yourself (and if you can truly enjoy the art of giving), then you are receiving twofold.

WHAT WE GIVE, WE RECEIVE

This comes when we understand that we are part of the one that consists of all. Awake is the consciousness to be aware of being part of God, the Creator of all. Your thoughts create everything, so when we learn how to control our thoughts we can make them work for us.

Everything that has ever happened in your life is the manifestation of your innermost desires, choices, ideas and concepts of who you are or choose to *be*. In 'being' you reveal who you think you are. By changing your concept of who you are, you change your 'being'. You are no longer the victim of your uncontrolled thoughts or the collective conspiracy that uses you as part of your karma. You can become the creator and make the collective consciousness your helpmate. On a large scale we all grow together; the more people we wake from unconsciousness, the more we will start giving freely to each other, the more we will shape what we all want – and that is to find happiness in being whole and complete.

Think back to the three levels of consciousness discussed in the Introduction to this book. We can see them now as the three levels of creation:

Level 1: your subconscious, uncontrolled thoughts, which create your reality.

Level 2: the collective consciousness, which, if you choose, can create your reality.

Level 3: your creative consciousness, which creates your reality in partnership with the collective consciousness.

And here is how you perceive these levels:

> **Level 1:** you try to gain control over what you have no control over. Things happen to you, which you put down to good luck or bad luck.

> **Level 2:** you try to adapt to what you have no control over. You become responsible for how you react to circumstances.

> **Level 3:** you become aware of the cosmic laws of manifestation and let the collective conspiracy work for you. 'You shape it until you become it.' The 'it' here is the one that consists of the many. You are a divine being and start to experience the larger, unified oneness and become part of this reality by choosing to stop creating your own individual reality. Now you are part of the effect of your choices. That is wisdom!

Next Paradox: Feeling Negative about Others Reveals the Negativity in You

One illusion many of us create is that others can *make* us feel a certain way. That is not true and not acceptable. Any time you feel negativity toward anyone, you are reliving part of your unresolved or suppressed emotions. The reality is that you have created this situation so you can heal a part of yourself. As such, you are the one in need of healing. Negative feelings create attachment, and attachment means you are not able to let go. If you cannot let go, you remain unconscious and unaware.

When we become dependent emotionally on others, we become enslaved by them. We are then in need of others' approval to be happy. This becomes a drug. We are not lonely due to lack of company; we are lonely because we are dependent on others to feel happy. The only reason you may not be perfectly happy right now is because you are focusing on what you *don't have* in your life right now. Your happiness is *conditional*. When you are in fear or worry or have any other emotion that is not released, it is because you believe something has been done to you.

These are some of the many things to which we devote our awareness, and they are without merit. We expend energy on areas that do not need our attention. We must learn to control these learned reflexes and focus our awareness on those things that do bring us harmony, peace, love and happiness. When we put negative thoughts or feelings in our mind, we are feeding it depleting and limiting stuff. This saps our life-force. We need to learn how to get control of our thoughts.

It is simple: if we focus on happy thoughts, we produce happiness in our mind. If our minds are happy, our cells are happy. If our cells are happy, we start regenerating and we get more vitality. When we focus on the sadness in our lives, we will be sad. Focus on enjoying life, on gratitude and God's love. These will erase negative emotions and allow us to have more life-force, more vitality and thus be caring, patient and more accepting of others. Spending time on the negative unresolved issues of our lives deprives us from being in the present. The 'present' is a present, a gift to ourselves. We have to live in the now. The most important moment in your life is right now. Start to feel happy and joyful right now. If you stop focusing on what you *don't have*, you will start experiencing the happiness of being given the present of now. Happiness comes from being free to choose, and being free makes you joyful and in balance. Ignorance causes fear. Not being aware of your incredible potential causes you to be afraid.

The Paradox of Death

So there are only two choices in life: love or ignorance. Either you understand this paradox or you don't. If you do not bring it into your life, you will stay fearful. How can you be fearful once you know you cannot die? Dying is actually liberation from all earthly worries. You are an immortal, infinite spirit having a limited human experience. You are not limited to your five senses. Your spirit is an observer; Deepak Chopra calls this the silent witness which never changes. It cannot change because it is part of the One Source most of us call God. The soul is the personal part of us that contains our intellect, memories, personality and the values of our higher consciousness. Your soul is the sum total of all your past feelings. Your soul can change and be cleansed of unresolved issues. Your spirit cannot die and your soul goes with it, with all its memories and unfinished business intact. Our physical bodies we can nourish with food, water and relaxation. Our soul and spirit are nurtured with love and compassion. These heal the soul and are the way to experiencing our ultimate being. Why should we fear death?

Understanding the paradox of death can liberate us from the biggest fear we have. When we are born, our spirit accepts the limitations of being human. When we die, we are liberated and experience ultimate freedom and bathe in the light of the Source of all life. We are returning to our spiritual home. By accepting this truth in our lives, we can stop making hell out of being alive, and stop fearing our transition to the place where we are free of all limitations. We came to this world to experience the limitations of matter and feel things like thirst and physical pleasures such as eating and sex. We can also experience things that are not common in the spirit world, such as anger, fear, hostility and sadness. As spirits we know only love. To define what love really is, we need to know what it is not. It is not greed, selfishness, cruelty, fear, worry, frustration and jealousy. Now we get to experience what love is not, so we can understand the true essence of the only source of life.

And so we come to understand that God does not punish us and that through the laws of karma we can cleanse the past and become our own healing force. So if there is something to learn here on Earth, it is that we need to follow our pure instincts. Our hearts, once calibrated to universal love, will guide us on how to nurture our souls. Having fear, anger or other emotions that consume you from within is not what you want. These feelings block your experience of feeling love, happiness and peace. By not letting negative emotions control you, you can release the hurt of the past.

You should use any encounter to reflect on where you are in your progress. By being aware of what goes on in your heart and not allowing negative emotions to blemish your soul, you can enjoy love at its purest, without fear. Emotions themselves are not negative or positive, though; it is their *effect* on us that counts. When people, despite our love and compassion, choose to go on with their actions, we can remove ourselves from their lives. We can love them from a distance where they have less effect on us. As we get healed and get stronger, fewer and fewer people can have a negative effect on our emotional state.

The Next Paradox: Your Life Is Exactly as You Want It to Be

Your life is the result of your unconscious desire. If you want something consciously, but you subconsciously believe you cannot have it, you will have what you consciously do not desire. Everything that happens on the outside comes from what happens within. The outside world is the reflection of your inside world. *What you are not aware of within you becomes aware outside of you.* What you are aware of, you can control; what you are not aware of will control you. When you are suffering it means you are out of touch with your divinity. When you awaken, you will understand the collective conspiracy. The driving force of Level 1 is to keep society in a coma. What is proclaimed 'normal' is false, meant to keep everyone wanting what they don't have. The main intention on this competitive level is to make a profit – but in the end we all lose. The planet is deteriorating because of our ignorance. We have become sheep who believe that if we can get more and more we'll be lions. The reality is that the more we buy into this illusion, the more we become unhappy and feel inadequate. We start believing we are failures because we are not as happy or beautiful as the people in magazines or on TV. Our role models are the rich and famous and those who have succeeded at Level 1, such as actors, athletes, politicians and musicians. Most of these people are, in fact, miserable.

THE QUESTIONS YOU WILL BE ASKED WHEN YOU GO BACK HOME

When we leave our body and are reborn in the spiritual realm, no one will ask us about our bank account or what car we drove. Nobody is interested in your test scores or how expensive your house was. What will be asked is whether you have succeeded in increasing your capacity to love and show compassion. If we have been successful in supporting those who were less lucky than us, how much would we have contributed to helping the cause of consciousness? So being rich and famous has nothing to do with being a success in life. When you awaken, you realize that it doesn't matter what others think of you. You realize that there is no need to worry about anything. The people who really make it are seldom front-page news; they are the silent ones. They don't pursue things that are worthless for their spiritual cause. They don't feel affected by the criticism of others nor their flattery or praise. It is the ego that fears there is not enough and needs external approval. No one can make you happy, because real happiness cannot be created outside of you. Happiness is your birthright and cannot be acquired.

HOW CAN I BE HAPPY?

The paradoxical answer to 'How can I be happy?' is that you have to let go of your false evidences and illusions. You are looking in the wrong direction. To be happy, you have to let go of the **F**alse **E**vidence **A**ppearing **R**eal (FEAR). When you let go of the illusions that cause fear, greed, ambition and craving more and more, you can enjoy your birthright.

When you buy an expensive car, you feel happy and thus have the evidence that happiness comes from stuff outside of you. You associate possessions with happiness. Sooner or later, however, you will discover that this is false evidence, because the ego will have new cravings, new fears, and so you have to buy something else to be happy. We have to unlearn all the hogwash we have been conditioned to believe. When you feel bad, that's because you have unresolved issues inside you. It's not your spouse, boss or others who are to blame. It is you!

Your first action is to stop blaming other people or outside circumstances for your suffering. You have to go inside to find the negative feelings. Remember, outside is the reflection of inside. Do not identify with these feelings, just observe them. You have to change; no one else has to change.

The most important paradox is that what we see is *just an illusion*. When someone rejects you or treats you badly, they are reacting to what they perceive you are. They are responding to an illusion created by their past unresolved emotions. They respond to the image which they project on you, based on their past. What they see is distorted by what they don't remember and do not know. So, the next time you feel rejected, remember that you can only feel rejected if you don't understand the workings of the minds of others. When you suffer, this points you to an unresolved part of yourself.

We have to learn to go through life without expectations. We can have preferences and opinions, but we cannot depend on them for happiness. We cannot judge others by what we see; we cannot judge at all, we can only observe. We know that we cannot trust our perceptions because these are coloured by the emotions we never have expressed or resolved. Reality is beyond knowing. We need to be able to observe what is going on within us and outside of us.

BECOME AWARE AND YOU ARE WHERE YOU ARE – THERE'S NO OTHER PLACE TO BE!

When we drop our opinions and judgements, we stop fighting over right and wrong. Spirituality is nothing less than awareness: the awareness that we need nothing and no one to be happy and the awareness that when we are not happy we are living in the past and not in the eternal now. If you do something you do not feel good about, this means you did it in an unconscious state. Once you open your eyes, you understand that freedom comes from living in your heart. When you seek the way of your heart, you lose your craving for external approval and success. Whatever you want for yourself, give it freely to others. The subconscious mind will believe you have abundance and create more of it. God bases your value in the future, not in the past. You can only be where you are right now, because now is the future and the past combined.

Just remember that life is about change. *The paradox is that you cannot change anything because you are already everything.* The only thing you can do is let go of those things that no longer serve you because you see through the illusion. Your concepts and ideas define who you are. Letting go of old concepts and beliefs redefines you. This accelerates your growth and spiritual evolution.

The three levels of consciousness amount to the following:

Level 1: your reality is created by your subconscious uncontrolled thoughts.

Level 2: you create your reality consciously by choice.

Level 3: you co-create your reality by serving the collective consciousness and letting it work for you.

When you reach Level 3, you submit to the universe and you become totally aware. You understand what universal love is. You understand that we are all related and that what you give to others, you give to yourself. You will be part of the One that is the Many, and not feel separate anymore.

THE PARADOX OF THE JOURNEY

There never was a journey to begin with; you have always been where you should be. The now is not a place to which you can travel. You can focus on the past, future or fantasy and not be aware of the now; this is Level 1 consciousness. Your happiness will be in the past, future or your fantasy. All possibilities come from the now; you have only to decide which possibility you want to embrace. Your purpose is to experience yourself. The journey we undertake is to stay in the eternal moment, the now. It's all too easy to get distracted and lose our focus. It's just like meditation. Meditation is a tool to help us learn to stay awake, to stay focused on the now. Then we get in touch with ourselves. The point and purpose of staying in the now is to choose who you really are and who you want to be.

The Next Paradox Is about Learning

We have nothing to learn; we already know. Our purpose is to remember that we already know.

You create the illusion we call life; do not become mesmerized by your own creation. Stay the observer and, if there are things you do not like, know that a part of you created them. Heal that part and create something you like.

To do this, to create something you like, you first have to accept what you don't like. You have to accept *all* of your creations. Talk to that part, discover its motivation and give it what it wants; that's acceptance without judgement. Judgement means rejecting that part of you. Do not deny or resist this part; if you do, it will only become rebellious and create more of what you don't like.

Another Paradox: in Silence Lie All Answers

By understanding this, you can grasp the concept that silence is the place where the soul will give you the answer. Daily meditation is one way to get in touch with your essence. In this way you will discover more of who you are.

One Is the Many

One is the source of All. The whole universe consists of one vibration which vibrates at different speeds, creating the illusion of the many. You cannot separate yourself from the Source. When you feel separated you have become brainwashed by your own illusion. You are not aware, you are in a coma. There is nothing to lose because there is a universal law that says that nothing can be lost; all there is will be all that ever is. What you give away you give to yourself because you are part of the whole. So, everything you do, you ultimately do for yourself. When another person makes you feel bad, it is because you make yourself feel bad. What is bad for another is also bad for you. All you are seeking in this world is already inside of you. Your heart is the temple where eternal love resides.

The Dog and the Bone

In Vedantic philosophy there is a saying: 'The joy of the world is like a bone to a dog.' The dog finds a bone and starts to gnaw on it. While he is gnawing on the bone, he gets splinters in his gums and they start to bleed. The dog tastes the blood and thinks, *This bone is delicious!* The more he gnaws on the bone, the more his gums bleed. The more blood he tastes, the more excited and happy he becomes.

This is an ongoing circle of self-realization. Just like the dog, we don't realize that what makes us happy comes from within. We use the outside world to access a feeling inside of us. That is why we have to find our own source within. To experience true happiness we have to focus our awareness on the inside. The paradox is that we have learned to look outside of ourselves for answers, while all the time they are within us.

DEATH IS YOUR ONLY GATEWAY TO HEAVEN

The greatest paradox of all is that you can only start living when you are not afraid to die. When you are ready to die, you start living. When you can live each moment as if it were your last, you have truly grasped the meaning of life. There is no routine anymore; everything reveals its beauty, everyone you see gives you joy, because you appreciate that this may be the last time you see them. You treat everyone with love and you forgive easily because you do not want to have any karmic debt. You realize that there is no time for negativity because that takes you away from enjoying the moment. Life is not about safety; it's a gamble and it's risky. Most people do not truly live because they seek security; people believe that living is about staying alive. It's the opposite: living is a dance with death. It's a deadly tango. Once you let go of the fear, you will enjoy the fluidity, the music, the movement and the rest of life. By accepting death as a friend rather than an enemy, you can focus on being alive and living fearlessly. Fear eats life energy and makes you a zombie, the living dead. Life is about letting go of your attachments and addictions, the need for approval or appreciation. You no longer depend on others to make you happy or miserable. It's about being, so take on activities that you can engage with your whole being. Love what you do and do what you love. Most people suffer not from the lack of love but from lack of awareness. We let ourselves down. We create deadlines, make demands on ourselves. Start to nurture your soul more, create time to get to know yourself: meditation, nature, music, Qigong, good books, good company. Stop feeding your interest in fame, power, wealth and attention. Otherwise you will become addicted to these sources outside of you.

Time to Journal

Journal your thoughts on the paradoxes mentioned so far, reading them again and making notes.

Steps Out of the Paradox-box

Step 1: be aware there is only now. When you are connected in the now, you feel love, harmony and peace, and you are optimistic. Any time you feel otherwise – miserable, angry, fearful – you are not connected to the Source. Go to Step 2.

Step 2: do not I-dentify, become an observer of the negativity. Realize it is inside of you and that the situation you've created is a chance for healing and reconnecting to the Source. As long as you think it's outside of you, you will leave the present. Accept the feeling and wonder at its sensations. You are experiencing the feeling, but you are not I-dentifying with it.

Step 3: accept and love yourself with the feeling and just let it be. After a short while it will fade away. Just like rain, it will stop and the sun will shine again.

These are three steps to emotional healing; we can access these with the approach we'll talk more about in the next chapters. But this is where it starts. We have to acknowledge that we are the creator of these feelings and that we are able to change them. Once we understand how this works, we can stay connected to the Source and experience love in all circumstances.

There will be many times when you will fail to follow these simple steps. Do not be too hard on yourself. Not many babies learn to walk gracefully in just a couple of weeks. This is a process that takes time to master. It's one of our priorities in life to master this process. Life only matters when you become good at it, when you can look death in the eye and smile. If you can do that, you can face any negativity. Everything else is easy compared to overcoming the fear of death. Be aware that most people can say intellectually they have no fears, but few can say it from their heart. That's the next step we will be working on: to become what we know.

Read the following summary at least 10 times to let all the information really sink in. There is so much in this chapter that goes against normal ideas and concepts that it will take repetition to change the limiting concepts you have in your mind.

SUMMARY

- There are no lessons to learn. We do not have to do anything; we just have to become conscious of how we make our choices.
- We are eagles believing ourselves to be chickens.
- To want something is to affirm you haven't got it. That's the best way not to get it.
- There is no past and there is no future; there is only the eternal now. The past is what you make of it, exactly as you create your future: *shape it until you make it.*
- Detachment from our creations makes us less dependent and more in control of our next creations.
- To change the now we have to change our thoughts.
- You have no free choice if you are not awake and aware. Our past is the perfect chosen way to serve our purpose to get to the now.
- We are here to find out why we are here.
- God is the 'I' of all there is and all there will ever be. 'I' am part of the total universal manifestation that is part of God.
- To be born is to die in another realm; to die is to be born again where you came from.

- The 'I' is the only constant there is; it's the silent witness.
- You can feel anger but you can never 'be' angry.
- You cannot label the 'I' nor put it in a box; the 'I' is the part that has no I-dentity and cannot be defined or described. It is I-nfinite and I-mmortal.
- To have something, you have to 'be' what it will give you first. If you can 'be' in the desired state, you will easily attract what you want – but, paradoxically, no longer need.
- Desire → desired state → attraction of desire.
- Happiness is a choice, not a result or outcome.
- Shape it until you become it (full sensory visualization: virtual reality).
- If you do not get what you want or if you get what you *don't* want, it means that part of you must want what you have got.
- Give to others what you desire most.
- The universe helps you to get more of what you feel.
- When we give we receive twice the amount, because we are part of the One that consists of all.
- Feeling negative about others reveals the negativity in you. All negative feelings create the opportunity to heal the past.
- The most important moment in your life is now, so you'd better enjoy it!
- Your soul and spirit are nurtured through love and compassion.
- Your life is exactly what you want it to be.
- Everything that happens on the outside comes from what is happening within. The outside world (macro-cosmos) is the reflection of your inner world (micro-cosmos).
- What you are not aware of on the inside becomes aware outside of you. What you are aware of you can control. What you are not aware of will control you.
- The main driving force of society is to keep you unaware.

Society wants you to believe you can be transformed from a sheep into a lion if you buy into its illusions.

- To be happy we have to let go of our False Evidence Appearing Real (FEAR is an illusion).
- When you feel bad it is because you are not aware of the unresolved issues within you.
- What we see is mere illusion; people react to their perceptions of you.
- Have no expectations, only preferences and opinions, but do not depend on them for your happiness.
- You cannot change anything because you are already everything; you can only let go of what no longer serves you.
- The highest level of creation is letting the collective consciousness do the work for you, effortlessly.
- There is no journey; we are always where we should be. There is no place to go except to the now and remembering what we already know.
- You cannot create freely if you do not first accept where you are and the part of you that shaped the now into what is.
- In silence lie all the answers of the soul.
- One is the many; you cannot be separated from the Source. Everything you do, you do for yourself.
- What makes us happy comes from within.
- You start living when you give up the fear of dying and live every moment as if it were your last.

Time to Journal

Write down your insights and which paradox you will focus on during the coming week, then change to another paradox until you have worked through them all.

CHAPTER 12

WWW.GOD...

Prayer of St Francis of Assisi

Lord, make me an instrument of your peace.
Where there is hatred, let me sow love;
where there is injury, pardon;
where there is doubt, faith;
where there is despair, hope;
where there is darkness, light;
and where there is sadness, joy.
Oh, Divine Master, grant that I may not so much seek
to be consoled as to console;
to be understood, as to understand;
to be loved, as to love.
For it is in giving that we receive;
it is in pardoning that we are pardoned;
and it is in dying that we are born to eternal life.

This chapter is a step into the Divine Self, to make you go deeper into the essence of who you are and what your purpose is. If I could summarize it in one sentence, it would be: *we are here to increase our capacity to love.* Because when we do, we come closer to ourselves. To understand this better we are going to embark on a fantasy trip. Let's play along in this chapter.

GOOGLING GOD

Imagine that God has a website. What keywords would you have to put in the search engine to find it? I would imagine words like 'universal love', 'unconditional love', 'compassion', 'forgiveness', 'heaven', 'peace', 'harmony', 'now', 'inspiration', 'truth', 'honesty', 'awareness', 'infinity', 'enlightenment'. What else can you think of? Perhaps 'guidance', 'angels', 'safety', 'eternity', 'source', 'life'. Let's imagine that we have logged onto this website. What would be on the home page?

GOD'S HOME PAGE

This is God, the source of all that is, all that was and all that ever will be. There is only good news to share with you; this website will guide you in a simple yet profound way to becoming more efficient at forgiving yourself and including yourself in my network of love, peace, harmony and compassion. By following these guidelines, you will master this little game I set up for you that you call life. The rules are simple: there is no right or wrong. You cannot get lost. There are no sins. Sins are illusions created by man. You are not your body and you cannot be harmed or insulted. You cannot die because you are immortal. What dies are your beliefs, ideas and concepts. You were never born; you have chosen to experience being human to understand what you really are. By finding out what you are not, you will know what you are. You are responsible for your actions and thoughts, and you are responsible for handling the actions and thoughts of others. You cannot make mistakes, you can only be aware of what you are conscious of. By being unaware, you create circumstances that will help you to become aware. You will experience feelings of rejection, loneliness, sadness, grief, anger, fear, worry, intransigence and insecurity to remind you that you are not aware. People will blame you as you will blame others for not being aware. You will judge others and they will judge you so you can show each other what you are not aware of. The most powerful tool that I can give you is the ability to remember that you are not aware.

You will project your fears and injustices on me, and believe I will punish you and send you to hell. This is the ultimate proof of your unawareness, because my love for you is the love for myself and I would never reject myself. Your thoughts and unresolved emotions are your worst enemies.

BECOMING YOUR OWN BEST FRIEND

You are your own worst enemy because you treat yourself worse than you would treat a dog; you believe you are worthless and deserve punishment for what you have done. Your real karma is the state of being unaware. By becoming aware, the past will dissipate instantly and you will be enlightened and embrace your shadow side (your human side). If you reject your human side, you condemn yourself – and others – and cast aspersions on all your accomplishments. By accepting and loving your shadow side, you are truly being human and your spirit can soar in the light.

FEAR IS A SIGN OF NOT BEING AWARE

Fear is the ultimate weapon that takes you out of awareness, followed by blaming yourself or others for your situations or feelings. Nothing is wrong and all circumstances are perfect for manifesting yourself. In this game called life you cannot lose because you are immortal. Nothing happens by accident or coincidence. Everything happens by agreement. All you see is a result of what you believe. Most of your beliefs are the beliefs of others based on the past. The rest of your beliefs come from your own past experiences. You are not guilty of anything. Just as someone who sleepwalks is not conscious of what he does, you are not conscious of who you are. You are sleepwalking. You have to wake up and come to terms with yourself.

All your negative feelings come from an unconscious feeling of guilt or shame. You are afraid that you are not loveable. Guilt and shame deny you a part of the beauty of one God. If you do not forgive yourself for feeling guilty or ashamed, you cannot become aware. You are your own judge; you have to become your own advocate who can help free you of being unaware. You are an eagle that thinks it is just a chicken and you refuse to wake up.

YOUR INNER DIVINE GPS

To lead you, I have given you a GPS (Global Positioning System) to show you the way home. This GPS is the voice of love and compassion; it will help you make the best choices in the maze of mirrors we call life. By asking the question, 'Does this bring me closer to experiencing more love?', you will get an answer from your heart. That will always be the right answer. You cannot go astray because at each turning point you will have guides and messengers. These guides and messengers will be disguised in many forms: words, street names, news items, brochures, books, angels, voices, etc. As long as you are aware, you will get the message. If that does not work, you may experience pain, suffering or disease. This is not a punishment but the result of having chosen paths that deplete your inner reservoirs of energy.

The highest betrayal is betraying yourself. You always have to love yourself first and do all you do without guilt or just to avoid punishment. All you give to another you give to God, and it will be given back to you. Do not give with the expectation of getting something back; see the other person as part of the All, and give freely. Everything you give will be returned with interest.

THE ULTIMATE GIFT

Forgiving is the ultimate gift; do not forget to give it to yourself. You profit through living in the awareness that you are giving to God even when you give to yourself. The only true means of control is by letting go and not seeking to control; then you are in control of your destiny. The only real security is not in possessions, but in not being possessed by anything. Obsession with security is the biggest insecurity there is. You are not separate from the whole, you are having your own customized experience. You customize your experience and through that you define yourself. If what you have created is not to your liking you are free to create something else. You can do this over and over until you master the process of creating what you like. As you grow, your tastes will change and you will start creating more ecologically and spiritually. You can create whatever you want, but if you don't love yourself you will not be happy with your creations. What you feel for others reflects what you feel for yourself. Excluding others from your love means you are excluding part of yourself from healing. Including them creates an opportunity for healing. To ask forgiveness from others is to become aware that you are no longer projecting your beliefs and fears onto others. Whether or not they forgive you is their choice and is irrelevant. If they don't forgive you, this shows only that they have more healing to do. Never do for another what he can do for himself; this will make him dependent on you and others, and keep him where he is. Also do not let another do what you have to do for yourself. Do not let others become the source of your happiness. Bless everyone in God's name; every time you bless someone, you are blessed. Show gratitude for all you have and all your experiences; do not focus on what you do not have.

BEING A VICTIM IS A CRIME AGAINST YOURSELF

All experiences are there to make you more aware of what is happening inside you. Are you a victim? That means you are not aware of why you attracted crime into your life; you are in danger of recreating it over and over again. This may happen in real life or in your mind. For your mind there is no difference between reality and imagination. By not letting go you are reliving and recreating the same circumstance over and over. Can you learn to turn being a victim into being a victor? Understanding the positive side or looking at the fear it brings out in you can heal the very part that attracted the event or situation in the first place. Accepting and loving that part of you jump-starts the healing process.

A LIFE EXPERIENCED FOR THE DIVINE

You are part of a big experiment; this experience allows God to experience what it is like to be human. All you do and all you experience is part of this experiment. You can at any time decide to create only what is to your liking, because that will be to God's liking.

Reconnection Is the Way to Go

In order to create what you like, you first have to really get to know yourself. You are much more than you believe you are. Your life's mission is to discover who you are by reconnecting with yourself. You can then create miracles and magic: in order to create magic in life you must be willing to let go of your limiting thoughts. Your limitations will determine what you create. God inspired Henry Ford to say the following: 'Whether you believe you can do a thing or not, you are right.' Shakespeare said it most eloquently, 'To be or not to be, that is the question.' Either you are or you are not. To be human is to discover what is it to be human; any box you put yourself into will be a limitation. The human experience is an experiment in integration, transformation and transcendence.

Integration of mind, spirit and body means having them work together as one. The spirit should be in charge because it's the highest form of being. When the mind or body dominates, we are not *being*, we are *doing* or *having*. By *being*, we don't have to do or have anything; we already are what we want to be. This is the most interesting riddle. Most people get it the wrong way round: they want something that is out of reach and associate it with a certain feeling (a form of being). Most people discover that feelings are temporary and, when those feelings are linked to external sources, part of the illusion we also call projection.

Transformation is the process of translating your mental and physical needs into soul-nourishing experiences instead of illusion-chasing ones.

Find the true intention of your needs and heal the soul, which is the wounded part of your spirit. It is wounded only because of its amnesia. Transformation is the process of curing amnesia of the soul and transforming the need. The need for approval comes from the belief you are not good enough. This is a miasmic belief. Understanding this, you no longer need approval and you can appreciate those who do not approve of you and see how they are projecting their own miasmic beliefs. You can help them transform and heal.

Transcendence is when you realize that the only things that matter are not from matter. Matter is the ultimate illusion. The source of all matter is what's important, and is the loving energy of creation. Transcending beyond the illusion of matter means you can still enjoy it without emotions of attachment, and you can dedicate yourself to the things that *do* matter: learning how to practise universal love, which is another word for compassion.

COMPASSION

Compassion is at the heart of all that matters, because it is the driving force of the universe. Seeking perfection is the affirmation of imperfectness. You should not seek perfection, because it is here already. You should become aware of the perfection in yourself and others. This will relieve your frustration at trying to be perfect. Just 'be' and all is perfect. You can use more of your potential to experience the situations you create and have the energy and intention to change and, in that way, create a completely new experience. Attachment to certain habits limits you to what you have already experienced and confines you to being a product of your past. By being so busy judging the situation, finding its imperfections and injuries and feeling miserable because it was not what you anticipated, you I-dentify with the negative feelings of the past and feel confirmed in what you are not.

You are at the centre of change. Your name stands for change. To be is to change. To be human is to create change. Every time you breathe or think, you change.

YOU ARE CHANGE

There are only temporary moments of imagined safety or security. Safety comes with accepting and welcoming change as a way of life. Living is the definition of change, so you had better be that change. The need for security recreates your past and enslaves you in a web of illusions that will cause you to close your eyes and become unconscious. Learn to smile at change, and learn to smile at people who change their mind. Congratulate them. Change is evidence of evolution: change your mind, change your thoughts and heal your soul. Do not try to trap others or yourself in the past. Do not dwell on the past or blame someone for past actions. A change of heart is the way to go. To feel memory and jump into the experience with an open heart, knowing that no one can really hurt you, is to know free choice. Pain is only the awareness of what needs healing. Free choice cannot happen if you are in the past and you lose your spiritual birthright. Growth means dying in the moment: what dies is the past, what's being born is the next moment.

Become a master at dying so you can stay in the present of life. To give meaning to something is to limit it; by living from your heart you demonstrate your emotional intelligence and ability to go beyond the limitations of what things might mean. Live fearlessly because you are immortal.

INTENTIONS AND LOVE FOR THOSE WHO ARE REJECTED

Tune in to the intention and be open for surprises. The only way to find out about someone's intentions is to open your heart and experience them. By opening up you can detach yourself and just be. What you don't like and does not feel right for you, let go of. Fall in love with being in love with all people. Truly open yourself to universal love without attachment; this is transcendence. 'Love people despite themselves;' most are not aware of who they are. The people who need love the most are those who reject it the most. Love without need for control or expecting something in return, with no conditions, no attachments. That is unconditional love, that is celestial love, that is connecting with the godhead. To connect with God or the Source, you have to learn to understand that all intentions are good. It is not intentions that create pain, it is how you *act on* your intentions.

IN REMEMBRANCE OF SADDAM HUSSEIN

Let's use Saddam Hussein as a prime example of someone who needed love and prayer. We all remember him; he paid dearly for his tyrannical ways. What he really wanted was love. He had learned that the only way to get attention was to provoke and control. He demanded attention; in his mind attention meant love. In my opinion it would have been better to have sent him love than killing him, which has created more chaos than anyone could have imagined.

Imagine the following: millions of people sending him loving postcards every week; he'd receive millions of them every week with loving thoughts. Not thoughts for change but simply letting him know that he was loved and that others were praying for his wellbeing. I know that Saddam would have been happy to know that so many people loved him, and he no longer would have needed to come up with all kinds of creative ideas to get attention. Even though he has left the planet he still needs to be loved so he can heal his soul and come back and do good for humanity. So include him in your prayers and send him love and compassion every day.

Some people who were very abusive in past lives come back to balance their deeds and to be anti-violence. Souls like Gandhi, Martin Luther King, Jr, Mother Teresa and many others might serve as examples. We all have been everything in the past, and we come back to balance our karma at some level.

GOOD AND BAD

You can create the world you want by seeing that there is nothing wrong with you or with anyone else. You have learned to polarize good and bad, and all of your fears come out of this. Society punishes those seen as bad instead of helping them to heal, instead of teaching them about love and instead of loving them. It releases them after confirming that they are bad, worthless and the scum of the Earth. Then something goes wrong in the equation: we expect them to behave differently. We control them for a while and, as long as they pretend to be healed and obey all the rules, we believe they are. This is insanity. We've only taught them more of the same. Most go right back to prison.

Our system of right and wrong does not function; instead of hiring more police and building more gaols, we need to invest more in solving the causes of this dis-ease of humanity. We have to create circumstances of equality through love and compassion. Ignorance is our worst enemy, after judgement and guilt.

Sharing your abundance with those who are born into limiting circumstances is sharing love and compassion. This is what spirituality is all about. Loving and sharing with the needy breaks the karmic chain. Believing that the needy are being punished for their negative karma creates your own negative karma, and robs you of the opportunity to heal yourself and the planet. If you have time to spare, get involved in community work. Giving is the biggest healing force in the universe after forgiving. There is no duality, no conflict, no choices to be made; there is only love and compassion. To connect with God is to see everyone as God's child and treat them the same as you wish to be treated.

The worst that can happen to someone is to be unaware that they are part of the Divine Source. They feel hurt, abandoned and rejected, and project their pain on the world. How often have you done the same? You are no better than anyone else. You may be less aware or more aware. There is no contest, everybody will get to the finish line and it isn't over until everybody makes it. By uniting you will only raise the collective consciousness and grow in your awareness. You can only judge the other when you are unaware yourself, as all judgement comes from fear, from isolating yourself from the Source. It is not a mistake to make a mistake. It will not take anything from you. You won't miss anything. It is only when you believe someone can take something from you that you will miss it and consider not having it a mistake. When there is an abundance of love, love cannot be taken, it is there **for** all to **get** – but we sometimes **forget**.

YOUR TRUTH

Accept your mistake of missing things and you will feel healed and forgiven. Perfection is the expression of truth without judgement and without any intention to hurt. The truth can heal, as long as you remember it is *your* truth. What's true for you may not be for another. Also, what you need to remember is that, as you inevitably change, what is true for you today may not be the same a moment from now. Remember that in the silence, you connect with your soul and you discover what needs healing. To become a good observer, you first need to learn to see what happens when you do nothing and just be. Through silence you connect with yourself and ultimately with God or the Source. Silence can be achieved through meditation and breathing. Listening to others and staying in the now is also a healing process. By observing yourself and what you feel, you can find which parts in yourself need healing. Become a good listener and observer and you will accelerate your own healing process.

Now let's focus on loving unconditionally. Be aware that the first person in line for healing is you, and that if you don't create the time and space for healing yourself, you cannot be fully of service to others. To learn unconditional love, you need to unlearn conditional love. Conditional love is based on others' belief that they depend on external sources to feel happy. They conditioned you to be a source of their happiness. A heavy responsibility was put on you. In order to make them happy, you had to deny yourself: you had to give up the love of self to make someone else feel loved. Most of us start believing this and it makes us condition others to do the same for us. When was the last time you heard something like: 'If you really loved me, you would…'? When we don't get this proof of love, we feel rejected, abandoned, unloved, worthless, insulted, not cared for, not supported or not accepted. Think about the last time something like this happened. What was the occasion? Go back to that moment and trace where it came from. Go back to your upbringing and look at your parents or teachers. How did they condition you to become dependent on their conditional love? How were they dependent on outside sources for their wellbeing? They were conditioned by their parents and they acted out what they had learned. They were conditioned by guilt, shame and a fear of not being good enough. Now it is up to you to release yourself, and others, from this karmic chain. It does not matter whether your parents or teachers are still alive; by breaking the chain you release all parties of karmic debt: that's what forgiveness is all about.

Your first next step in the healing process is to give yourself what you've never had: unconditional love. It is up to you, nobody else. If you do not do it, nobody else will. God already loves you unconditionally, no strings attached. Now you have to follow suit.

Time to Journal

Write down your insights and how you can love more, and to whom you can show more appreciation and gratitude.

SOUL-WORK

Your soul is the part that needs healing. Your soul is wounded by old experiences which no longer serve you. The biggest fear your soul can come up with is, 'What if all of this isn't true? What if God does not love me? What if I am not worthy?' All these questions are the products of fear; you need to detach yourself from them by accepting them and loving the part of you that is fearful. So, do not ignore these thoughts but acknowledge them. Here is a way that will accelerate your healing tremendously. Do this at least twice a day for a minimum of four weeks and you will experience a big change in your heart. The more often you can do it, the better.

Twice a day, stand in front of the mirror, look yourself in the eye and massage the acupoints for fear (see page 147) with one hand while you say:

- 'I accept and deeply love myself with my fear of not being worthy of God's love.'
- 'I deeply accept and love my fear of not being worthy.'
- 'I love myself and accept myself, even when I do not feel worthy or not loved or rejected.'
- 'I accept and love myself even if this fear will never go away and give my soul permission to let go completely and permanently of this fear.'

This is the foundation for emotional healing. It's not about being fearless; it's about accepting and loving yourself with your fear. Accept and love those parts of you that still need this fear. Write these affirmations down on a piece of paper and carry them with you everywhere. When you are irritated, frustrated, angry or worried and you realize that this is coming from you, and that all negative emotions come from fear, you can repeat these affirmations while stimulating the fear acupoints. You can also customize the affirmations; for example: 'I accept and deeply love myself with my frustration which comes from my fear of not being good enough.'

You cannot go wrong; there is nothing you can do or say to yourself to make things worse. Finish off each sentence with the following (using the fear acupoints): 'I unconditionally accept and love myself and I am fully worthy of God's unconditional love, now and continuously.'

What you will discover is that when you awaken out of the illusion of conditional love and start giving yourself unconditional love, you will attract others who will do the same. The more you own these affirmations, the less needy you become; you will become self-supporting and self-loving, and as a result you will be able to give freely to others. You become less and less controlling and will eventually refrain from making others dependent on your love or approval. You will become aware of the growing universal love in you, and start to see the godlike in everyone.

Once we make the transition from judgement to acceptance we open our hearts for compassion. It all starts with loving yourself. So stop judging yourself and start accepting you, in your totality. At first it will feel impossible to stop judging; the more you focus on not judging, the more you will judge yourself and others. You may start to feel guilt. The way to break through this is to accept that you judge and forgive yourself for that. Just observe that a part of you still needs that; accept and love that part. Thank this part of you for its good intentions. It is the same with fear: accept it, love it, play with it until you transform it.

Believing you are less than you are is a manifestation of fear. Accept your limiting thoughts without trying to change them. Just observe, send love and let go. Acceptance is the first step of healing. There is nothing wrong with you. All is exactly as it should be. We are on track with evolution and everything is going according to plan.

Any pain or fear is a part of you asking for healing. Every mistake you make is a chance to learn something about yourself, so cherish your mistakes and be thankful for the lesson. Come out of denial and become one with what you feel. Let your soul speak truthfully through you by acknowledging your feelings and expressing them openly. Become aware of your thoughts and observe and acknowledge them; let them be, they will take care of themselves.

Feelings of being victimized are part of your old beliefs; accept that you used this as a tool to manipulate yourself and others to get love, empathy, attention and compassion. Give those things to yourself freely without needing to play the victim. Being a victim only brings you the opposite of what you want, and will lead to you believing that you do not deserve love. Give love to those parts that are wounded and are unforgiving, heal them and you will feel better. Remember to be aware of all that you are thankful for; show your gratitude by sharing your abundance with others who are less fortunate. Gratitude is the awareness of the universal blessing. Receive all the gifts you get with gratitude and let go of negativity about what you receive. Become totally defenceless, do not justify your opinion, accept the opinion of others and respect them for sharing. See the God in everyone and become part of the healing, not part of the dis-ease.

WE ARE ALL ONE

Spirituality has everything to do with understanding that we are all one. To have abundance and not share is to confirm your scarcity and lack of awareness. As long as there is discrimination and some people believe they are more worthy, more evolved or more spiritual or more right than others, there is a lack of integration. When you learn to love those who oppose you, you will have made a lot of progress. When you learn to choose according to your compassion, you are aware. Spiritual leaders will not show you the way but will give you the tools so you can discover your own path. Love those who try to manipulate you but choose not to be made complicit in their lack of love for themselves.

Many parents manipulate their children by trying to make them feel guilty. Many children feel guilty or angry and yet still do what the parents want. You can love your parents without letting them manipulate you. Their blame or accusations are expressions of their conditioning and pain. Pray for them, show compassion and be patient. Forgive and give what you can without guilt, from your heart. When you feel attacked, do not go in defensive mode but become vulnerable and feel the other's pain; send out love and compassion, make all choices from your heart. The other person is asking for your love in the only way he knows how.

Remember to use the gift of forgiving as much as possible; each time you forgive, you break karmic chains and you experience the glory of God. Forgiveness is the gift that multiplies manyfold. Forgiveness is connecting with the source of unconditional love, it's the mother of all healing, it's the beacon that will bring you back to the Source. Forgiveness is the best tool for emotional balance and leads you to spiritual intelligence. It clears your heart and heals your soul. Forgive every day, especially yourself and all those you believe have caused you any harm.

UNIVERSAL LOVE AS HEALING

Love is the most powerful tool that we are given to do healing; there is nothing more effective than love. The secret is to give it to others universally. It will open you to a new awareness of being alive.

Make Your Love Felt

Choose your words, intonation and attitude carefully, and use your eyes, face and body to express what you feel inside. When you start practising universal love and putting your focus on it, you will find the world responsive. Show interest in others and encourage them; show them respect, gentleness and, most of all, compassion. Do things that no one expects of you. Buy hundreds of beautiful postcards and send them each week to a few people whose hearts you want to touch. Surprise relatives with flowers, ring people you don't normally speak to a lot and let them know you care. Who are the people you have let fade out of your life? Make a list of all the people you know and think of actions you can do to let them know you care. Not because you want their love but because you want to practise universal love. Pay attention, be aware of the people who serve you, find something you genuinely like about them and tell them. Make them feel good, without wanting anything in return. Express your love to your spouse, your children and all your close and distant relatives. Also, show your concern for colleagues, people who work with you or for you. Make this a habit every day.

Once in a While, Do Something Extraordinary

Smile more and look people in the eye, acknowledge them and let them know their efforts are appreciated. Find the good in everyone; if there are things you want them to do differently, tell them first what is good about how they're doing and then tell them what you think needs improvement. Keep that part short, do not judge, do not criticize and do not let it come between you. Finish with something positive or encouraging. Be kind, gentle and respectful to everyone, even those who don't treat you this way in return. Work on this every day from now on. If one day things don't go the way you want, start over again the next. Soon this will become a habit, you will show love to everyone and feel good about it. Do not suppress anything, stay honest with yourself, this is not an act; it's connecting with the Source of all.

Last but Most Important Step

Every day, do a random act of kindness. That means looking around you and, whenever you see someone that you resonate with (positive or otherwise), approach this person, say something nice, offer your help and be kind to them. Mahatma Gandhi said, 'My love burns hot, but if there is still suffering in my world, my love does not burn hot enough!' That is a beautiful example of how to take responsibility for all that is around you and to step into the power of action and help to be part of the change you want to see.

Thank you for visiting this website. If need be, come visit this website again; you will discover new information each time, and repetition is the mother of all skills.

Be blessed and find peace in your heart.

Man's best friend for eternity: God.

CHAPTER 13

LET THE HEALING BEGIN

In the previous chapters we've talked at length about emotional healing. In this chapter you will get some tools to start your own healing process.

Time to Journal

If you really want to heal, you must deal with the major issues in your life:

- fear of death
- fear of not being worthy of love
- beliefs that others can hurt you or reject you
- guilt for things you've done
- shame or feeling victimized
- traumas from the past
- feeling unforgiving or being afraid to let go
- feeling the need to control.

Complete the list of things you want to heal in your life. Use extra paper if needed. We will get back to this later when you have the tools. Write them down now and do not continue reading until you've spent at least 15 minutes on this task.

STRESS ELIMINATION

To heal means to eliminate all the stressors in your life by healing the parts of you that experience stress. *Stress is not what happens but the meaning we give to what happens.* To become aware of stress you have to become aware of what's happening inside you. When you do not feel peaceful, loving or in harmony you are stressed and you need to do some healing. Remember, you want to observe the feelings and not I-dentify with them. Just let them be and then move on to acceptance and the healing mantra we will explore together shortly.

It is important to become aware of your feelings and your thoughts. By observing your actions and what you say, you will gain even more information. Awareness of healing means learning to know when anything threatens to take you out of harmony (your still-point). When you feel anything that causes discomfort, either inside or outside of you, it is an indication of a part of you that needs healing. For example: you are in a traffic jam and someone illegally cuts you off. Do you feel anger or frustration? There are many events in life where we feel justified in being upset, insulted, angry, frustrated or irritated. These feelings come from our soul which needs healing. When you get cheated and taken advantage of, you will feel very bad, very upset. Everyone will agree with you: you *should* feel that way. Nothing is further from the truth. When you have evolved you will not feel offended, you will forgive and break the karmic chain.

Here is another familiar situation: someone shows up late to meet you and you feel upset. You may think they do not respect you, especially if they do not apologize. Start paying attention to the situations in which you feel justified in feeling a certain way; when you are certain you are right and the other person wrong or impolite or rude.

There are many places to begin with healing. I have been working diligently on this for the last two years and there are not many things left that can disturb my balance. I feel incredibly happy most of the time and my relationships are more open, honest and stress-free. I do not care what people think of me, and my self-esteem has shot up tremendously. I have been attracting new people into my life. I have connected with some wonderful people. I am doing much more than ever before with less effort, and I feel blessed.

Some of the people I have been working with have changed my life. I have heard similar stories from thousands of people doing my seminars or attending workshops run by other instructors or working with practitioners of Omega Healing (more about this on page 60). You have to become conscious of what you are feeling and what your thoughts are in order to heal your soul completely. Anybody can learn how to do this. Feelings are fuelled and given a charge by unresolved issues. Healing consists of different elements:

1. A healing formula to assist your subconscious mind in finding the first incident that caused the unresolved chain of emotions.
2. Specific acupoints that will balance the meridians to speed up the healing process.
3. Specific breathing exercises to integrate the process in the chakras and neurological system.

This healing technique has been developed using different elements from different disciplines, acupuncture and affirmations. It has been field-tested on more than 20,000 people to verify its efficacy. The results are beyond any other simple technique I've studied over the past 20 years. This combined technique is called the *Emotional Healing Formula*; it is part of emotional balance. The most beautiful aspect is that you can do it all by yourself and do not need another to assist you. This gives you the means to use it anywhere and you can share it with anyone. You will get to know where you are hurt and how to heal yourself. You do not need psychoanalysis because your subconscious mind knows everything there is to know. You can also use the Omega Healing sessions (12 guided meditations) to guide you through this process – check page 288 for more information.

Emotional balance is used by thousands of people in Europe and has been taught in over 20 countries. The Emotional Healing Formula will connect you with your soul and your spirit, and bring you back to your true essence. It will connect you with the Source of all. You do not have to be religious to use this formula. Do not let the words distract you or trigger a negative response in you; this is universal and not meant to discomfort anyone. If you believe in

angels, the messengers of God's love, you can ask them to assist
you and guide your healing. The word 'angels' comes from ancient
Aramaic and is best translated as *messengers* (see Nick Bunick's book
In God's Truth). These messengers, or guides, are always with us;
they support us in our spiritual evolution and remind us that only
when we are in harmony with what is inside us, with our spirit or
Higher Self, the 'I', can we find unconditional happiness. Make use
of your angels as much as possible; this will speed up your healing
and help you to find inner peace.

Emotional Healing Formula
During the processing of your feelings, you massage the
acupoints for fear (next to the breastbone, under the
clavicle) and say:
'I accept myself and deeply love myself with my fear of
letting go of this feeling. I accept myself even if I will never
let go of this feeling completely.'
(Inhale and exhale deeply) → *Focus on chakra 1: flexibility*
(If you accept the belief in angels, you can say the following):
'I ask my angels and guides to assist me to the origin of this
feeling (or thought) of …, however long ago, and help me to
heal this completely.'
(Inhale and exhale deeply) → *Focus on chakra 2: enjoyment*
(If you do not want to work with angels, you say): 'I ask my
spirit (or Higher Self) to go back to the very first time I ever
experienced this feeling (or thought) of …'
(Inhale and exhale deeply) → *Focus on chakra 2: enjoyment*
'I allow every part and aspect of my being to assist me
to heal this original incident, however long ago, and to
completely accept and love the original intention.'
(Inhale and exhale deeply) → *Focus on chakra 3: acceptance
and letting go*
'I forgive myself, by the love of God, for rejecting myself
and others, for my incorrect beliefs, thoughts, feelings and
perceptions, and I forgive any person, incident, others and
anything involved, and let go of any reason or belief to

need this any longer or at any time during any of my past experiences. I allow the healing to be complete for all related incidents ever since.'

(Inhale and exhale deeply) → Focus on chakra 4: peace and forgiveness

'I now let go and release with unconditional love and God's blessing all of the old that was part of my feeling or thinking this way, now and continuously. I choose to replace this with ... *(positive feelings or thoughts)*. I accept this feeling of ... *(positive feeling)* in every cell of my body.'

(Inhale and exhale deeply) → Focus on chakra 5: expressing yourself truthfully

'I am giving myself permission to let go of any related discomfort on a physical, emotional, mental and spiritual level, or any related attitude, behaviour or feelings with ease and grace, now and continuously.'

(Inhale and exhale deeply) → Focus on chakra 6: knowing yourself

'I thank God, my guides and angels (or Higher Self) for all their help, and express to them my love and gratitude. I accept and am worthy of all of God's blessings and love.'

(Inhale and exhale deeply) → Focus on chakra 7: universal love

The positive feelings with which you replace the negative feelings are important. Do not let this be an intellectual exercise; it is important to really feel these emotions in your body. Allow your body to express what's in your mind, and then allow this feeling to go to every cell of your body.

Visualize this feeling moving through your body as if it were light, illuminating every cell.

Breathing: in total there are seven times when you will breathe deeply in and out. Each time you will connect subconsciously with one of the chakras and bring the energy higher into your system. It's best to focus on the specific area related to each chakra as you do this and imagine a warm feeling in this area.

Chakra 1	Base of your coccyx
Chakra 2	Around the area of your pubic bone
Chakra 3	Solar plexus or navel
Chakra 4	Around the area of your heart
Chakra 5	Your throat area
Chakra 6	Between your eyebrows (third eye)
Chakra 7	Just above your head (1 or 2 inches/2.5 to 5 cm)

Just bring your attention to the chakra area. You can also connect the chakras with specific feelings. Do not worry about this too much at the beginning. As the Emotional Healing Formula becomes more of a routine, this will become easier.

Chakra 1	Flexibility (adapting to all challenges)
Chakra 2	Enjoyment of life (enjoying the process of life)
Chakra 3	Accepting and letting go (letting go easily)
Chakra 4	Peace and forgiveness (harmony)
Chakra 5	Expressing yourself truthfully (not holding back your feelings)
Chakra 6	Knowing yourself (listening to your inner voice and guides)
Chakra 7	Universal love (tapping the collective Oneness)

The breathing goes as follows: take a deep breath through your nose as fast and deeply as possible, hold the breath for a few seconds, relax, close your eyes and, while focusing on the specific chakra, the specific keywords and the feelings, slowly exhale through your mouth, imagining that you are breathing through your chakra. Meanwhile you are massaging the acupoints for fear.

Healing can happen in an instant when we are ready. Most of the time healing is a gradual process. This is because most of us need time to change our thoughts, ideas and views. This takes time.

As you make this a routine in your life and use the Emotional Healing Formula on a daily basis, you become more and more balanced. It will be easier and easier for you to stay at still-point. You will become more and more focused on the positive feelings that are deep inside of you. It is important to find positive feelings to replace the old feelings; this can be done with just a word or with complete sentences. It does not matter as long as you allow that feeling to be inside of you. By using the chakra-keywords and focusing on those feelings, you are accelerating the healing process tremendously. If you do not find an appropriate feeling to replace the old one, it is always good to use unconditional happiness and harmony.

The Emotional Healing Formula connects us immediately with the 'I' and the source of all: God. It is not embracing one religion over another; it is your own direct prayer for healing and utilizes all parts of your soul and Higher Self to connect to God's unconditional love. It will immediately raise your vibrations to a positive level of love, peace and harmony, which is the spiritual level of healing. You are going directly to the level of anti-matter, the so-called holographic blueprint, and you are unifying all systems together: your energetic body, mind, soul and spirit, the most powerful healing combination known to humanity.

The Emotional Healing Formula will do far more than create emotional balance. When you follow the ideas behind it, you will be able to heal yourself at all levels. It will bring you, step by step, to Level 3 of manifestation and help you to live *chosaku*, letting go and resolving most of your negative karma. *Chosaku* is a Japanese word indicating that you are not creating new negative karma, but burning old negative karma. It is conscious living with the intent to cleanse your soul and liberate your spirit. You will become more and more in tune with God's loving will and use your heart as your compass and enjoy life to its fullest. Listening to your heart will also guide you to the path where there is no need for dis-ease. It is the path of least resistance. Dis-ease can also be healed faster by applying the Emotional Healing Formula. Remember not to fight the dis-ease but to accept it as your own creation, a way for your subconscious to let your attention remind you of an area in your life that needs healing.

Major areas to work on (soul-cleansing):

- I am worthy of being loved.
- I accept and love myself at the deepest level.

- I accept and am at peace with the fact that I will die one day.
- I let go of all guilt and shame.
- I forgive myself completely for all past mistakes.
- I forgive all other people for what I feel that they have done to me.
- I am totally committed to living consciously and allow God's love into my life.

You can make these more specific, for example: 'I am worthy of being loved despite the fact that my father gave me the impression he did not love me.'

- 'I accept and love myself at the deepest level and I am committed to stopping self-destructive habits [smoking, drinking].'
- 'I accept and I am at peace with my fear of dying.'
- 'I accept my difficulty in letting go of my guilt/shame.'

I would recommend you prioritize the areas of importance and start with those that are your highest priority. Commit yourself to working on these areas daily for the coming months and add whatever triggers you on a day-to-day basis. If you meditate, do this before your meditation; this will benefit your meditation tremendously and you will get more out of it. I also recommend you start practising Qigong. If you do, I'd advise that it's best to do this exercise first.

As with meditation or Qigong, it is important to use this Emotional Healing Formula in a comfortable, preferably quiet place. Make it special if at all possible. Light a candle and find an aromatherapy fragrance that you like, or incense, and put on some comforting music. Sit down and relax. Close your eyes and breathe in and out slowly. Then focus one by one on your seven chakras. Use the seven words related with the chakras and tune in to the corresponding feelings:

- flexibility
- enjoyment of life
- accepting and letting go
- peace and forgiveness
- expressing the self truthfully
- knowing the self
- universal love.

Then, I would also invite angels and guides to come closer, to support and assist your healing. With your eyes closed, imagine being surrounded by loving beings of light that come to support you and assist you to heal your soul. They are always close by and ready to help. Now you are ready to start the deep healing. Let's say you are working on this issue: 'I am worthy of being loved.' This is how you could do it.

Start by massaging the acupoints for fear (next to the breastbone, under the clavicle); then say the following: 'I accept and deeply love myself with my fear of letting go of this belief of not being worthy of being loved. I accept myself even if I will never let go of this belief completely.'
Inhale in deeply (fast) – exhale slowly and bring your attention to the area of chakra 1 (just above the tip of the coccyx). Focus on feeling flexible, ready to adapt to all challenges. Feel safe and secure, knowing you can handle anything that happens in your life. Breathe as if you are breathing through this area.
'I ask my angels and guides to assist me to go to the origin of this belief, however long ago, of not being worthy enough to be loved and help me to heal this completely.'
and/or
'I ask my spirit (or Higher Self) to go back to the very first time I ever experienced this belief of not being worthy enough of love.'
Inhale deeply (fast) – exhale slowly and bring your attention to the area of chakra 2. Imagine breathing through this area

around your pubic bone. Focus on feeling joy, pleasure and gratitude for all the good things in your life.

Continue with (while massaging the acupoints for fear):
'I allow every part and aspect of my being to assist me to heal this original incident, however long ago, and to completely accept and love the original intention.'

Inhale deeply (fast) – exhale slowly and bring your awareness to the area of chakra 3 (around the navel or solar plexus) and imagine breathing through this area. Focus on feeling open and receptive (accepting) and able to let go of the past gracefully. Imagine the past dissolving and disappearing through this chakra.

'I forgive myself by the love of God for rejecting myself and others for my incorrect beliefs, thoughts, feelings and perceptions, and forgive any person, incident, others and anything involved and let go of any reason for believing I need this any longer or during any of my past experiences. I allow the healing to be complete and to extend to all related incidents ever since.'

Inhale deeply (fast) – exhale slowly and bring your awareness to the area of chakra 4 (around your heart) and imagine breathing through this area. Focus on feeling peaceful, loving and forgiving and promise yourself to open your heart completely to let go of all past traumas. Imagine how your emotional scar tissues disappear through forgiveness and the unconditional love of God.

'I now let go and release with unconditional love and God's blessing all the old feelings that were causing me to feel or think this way, now and continuously. I choose to replace this with feelings of being worthy of love and self-esteem. I accept this feeling of being valuable and worthy in every cell of my body.'

Inhale deeply (fast) – exhale slowly and bring your focus to the area of chakra 5 (around your throat) and imagine bringing light and energy to this area. Focus on feeling at ease, expressing your innermost feelings and thoughts truthfully. Imagine this light or energy spreading through your whole body and feel full of God's love and appreciation. Bring this to every cell in your body and fill them with this light until you see yourself as one big source of light.

Continue now with:

'I am giving myself permission to let go of any related discomfort on a physical, emotional, mental and spiritual level, or any related attitude, behaviour or feelings, with ease and grace, now and continuously.'

Inhale deeply (fast) – exhale slowly and bring your focus to the area of chakra 6 (between your eyebrows) and imagine bringing light that you inhale into this area. Focus now on opening yourself up to the guidance of your Higher Self, spiritual guides and angels. Imagine seeing these guides and angels, receiving messages from them that will help and assist you on your spiritual path.

Finish with:

'I thank God, my guides and angels (or Higher Self) for all of their help and express to them my love and gratitude. I accept and am worthy of all of God's blessings and love.'

Inhale deeply (fast) – exhale slowly and bring your essence of your being to the area of chakra 7 (just an inch or two above your head) and imagine a beam of light connecting you with the source of all life and feel God's unconditional love and compassion for you and all beings. Let this light fill you up from head to toe with truth and hope and feel connected with the universe.

Return now to your body and feel your body. When you feel like it, open your eyes.

How does it feel to try this Emotional Healing Formula? Be aware of how powerful this is and, each time you do it, you will find it even more powerful due to the accumulated effect. Work with the same issue at least 21 times to get the full effect. You can work on several issues one after another, but do not overdo it. Allow your body to adjust.

Write the formula down and carry it with you everywhere you go. Use it as often as you want. Also continue reading for more tips on how to speed up your healing and become emotionally balanced. The formula cleanses the soul and resonates with your spiritual DNA. Your spiritual DNA is your soul's purpose for being, the original plan of why you are here. This practice will help you to get in touch with that, especially when you combine it with meditation or Qigong.

MORE TIPS AND TOOLS

There are five categories that are related to unresolved emotions or feelings. Analyzing these categories helps you get more out of your Emotional Healing sessions:

1. Mental thoughts, beliefs, ideas, images, memories
2. Attitude behaviour (physiology, voice, composure)
3. Incidents stress (traumas, people, environment)
4. Feelings emotions, sensations, moods, pain
5. Physical sensations pain, disease, cravings

These five categories are interrelated and influence one another.

There is one more category that is more difficult to define: spirituality. This relates more to unease stemming from not being on the right path (not following your *dharma*, the path of magic, of bliss and effortlessness). Unhappiness, restlessness and accidents can be the result. For simplicity, I will not bring this one into the picture right now, but you can add it if you feel comfortable with it.

When we change in one of these categories, all the other ones are affected as well. Changing your beliefs has a tremendous impact on your attitude, stress levels, feelings and physical body. Now is a good time to reread the chapter www.God... This can change your life.

Let's have a look at an example.

Harry was a bright eight-year-old. His mother brought him to see me because he was forgetful and tired all the time. Not a day would pass by without Harry forgetting something somewhere, from his lunchbox to his clothes or shoes. He was also unable to remember anything that happened in school. Strangely enough, he always got good marks on tests. Harry looked at me with his big sky-blue eyes and I saw his despair and sadness. I asked him what he could tell me about school that day. 'We played outside,' he told me. 'Anything else?' I asked. 'We were in class all day!' Whatever I asked, he could not get more specific than that. He said, 'I have a bad memory, I keep forgetting things!' I asked him why he said that and he replied, 'Everybody tells me that.' I told him that others were completely wrong, and that he had a great memory, while I showed him all the things he remembered: how to do maths, how to speak, how to dress, how to play basketball, football, monopoly, draughts, chess and so on. 'Harry, do you know there is not one computer in the whole wide world that can do as many things as you can?' Harry's whole physiology changed: he smiled, sat up straight and looked at his mum to see if she were listening.

I showed Harry how to massage the acupoint for self-esteem, and explained to him that this was a magic secret way to enhance memory, and that he had to massage it at least three times a day while saying, 'I have a great memory; I remember everything easily.'

Here is how Harry's 'five categories' looked before he came to see me:

1. Mental   he believed he had a terrible memory; this was constantly confirmed by others.

2. Attitude   low self-esteem and apologetic

3. Incidents   stress at home and at school, because he could not find anything and forgot things

4. Feelings   of inadequacy: 'I am worthless.'

5. Physical   exhaustion, low energy

Two weeks later Harry was a completely different boy. The puffiness under his eyes was gone, he was not forgetful anymore, he felt great and freer than ever before.

This kind of situation happens all the time: we focus on our weaknesses, help others focus on theirs, and get stuck in that mode and cannot get out anymore. We should focus on how to help and support others.

Here is another example.

Mary, a 26-year-old woman, is an alcoholic and suffers from depression. She is suicidal and does not want to live anymore. She does not believe that she is worthy of having a good relationship and feels she is a failure. She sits for hours in front of the TV, snacks a lot and is on Prozac.

Six months ago her fiancé told her, just three weeks before the wedding, that he was in love with another woman. This woman, he said, was his soulmate and they were destined to be together. He left Mary. She was devastated, and also mortified at having to call the wedding off. This had been her second relationship and had lasted for four years; her previous relationship had ended after three years. She gained 10 pounds and got fired for coming in late and not being able to finish her tasks. That's when she began drinking.

Let's look at Mary's 'five categories':

Mental	'I am a failure, nobody loves me.' Recurring thoughts of suicide. Also, she remembered that her father never said he loved her. 'I am worthless.'
Attitude	depressed, does not speak up or at times very rebellious and angry
Incidents	wedding cancellation, father who did not express his emotions
Feelings	'who cares?' – despondency, despair
Physical	cravings for alcohol, snacks, excessive sleep

The areas we focused on in healing were changing Mary's beliefs about herself and to remind her of the events and people in her life that were proof she was loved. Her mother had always expressed her love. Gradually we changed her feelings about herself, and her cravings for sugar and alcohol disappeared as well.

It is always important to create a supportive environment for healing and to remove yourself from people who will block your healing and growth.

DAILY USE OF THE EMOTIONAL HEALING FORMULA

Use the Emotional Healing Formula (see page 253) any time you feel uncomfortable, stressed, angry, upset or frustrated. Always remember that the external triggers (incidents) only have an effect if something inside needs healing. Scan your beliefs, attitude, physical sensations and emotions, and after the session experience how this has changed. The incident or trigger should no longer throw you off. If it still does, this only means you need to do it more often until you reach complete still-point. Still-point means you feel peaceful and at ease when you think of the situation or when you are in it again. A good way is to grade your level of discomfort from zero to 10, with zero being completely at ease and peaceful and 10 being the worst possible intensity of emotion you can imagine. After the healing session, grade the intensity again; there should be a difference now. If there is no difference, you should try the technique for emotional reversal.

Make a fist with one hand and start hitting (gently) the palm of the other hand. After five or six hits, alternate the hands. Speed it up until you can do this as fast as you can.
Now say the following sentences:
'I accept and love myself at the deepest level even if I will never be completely happy, healthy and successful.'
Inhale deeply (fast) and exhale more slowly, then proceed
'I accept and love myself at the deepest level even when I

will become extremely happy, healthy and successful.'
Inhale deeply (fast) – exhale more slowly and proceed
'I accept and love myself at the deepest level even if I will
never let go of this feeling/thought/belief of … (fill in what
you are working on now).'
Inhale deeply (fast) – exhale more slowly and continue
'I accept and love myself at the deepest level even if I will
let go of this feeling/thought/belief of … (fill in what you are
working on now).'
Inhale deeply (fast) – exhale more slowly and continue
'I accept and love myself at the deepest level even if I am not
willing to let go completely of this feeling/thought/belief
of … (fill in what you are working on now) and would like to
keep some of it.'
Inhale deeply (fast) – exhale more slowly and proceed
'I accept myself and love myself at the deepest level and
I feel completely comfortable to let go of this feeling/
thought/belief of … (fill in what you are currently working
on) completely and permanently **now**.'
Inhale deeply (fast) – exhale more slowly and proceed
'I accept and love myself at the deepest level even if I still
have reasons, beliefs or parts of me that will resist my letting
go of this feeling/belief/thought of (fill in what you are
currently working on) **now**.'
Inhale deeply (fast) – exhale more slowly and continue
'I accept and love myself at the deepest level possible even
when I let go and heal all reasons, beliefs or parts of me that
were resisting the complete and permanent letting go of
this feeling/thought/belief of … (fill in what you are currently
working on) **now**.'
*Inhale deeply (fast) – exhale more slowly and you can stop
making a fist now.*

After a session you will have eliminated most of the hidden
saboteurs to your healing. Now go back and repeat your Emotional
Healing Formula (see page 253).

You can also routinely practise emotional reversal (see page 264).

What we achieve with the alternating movement of the fists and the breathing is:

- equalizing the information in the left and right brain
- stimulating the specific acupoints for the small intestine meridian, which helps to create emotional balance and integrates unresolved emotions
- accessing the limbic system, which contains the emotional hologram (blueprint) of all unresolved emotions.

The faster we do this, the more we engage the neurological system; the affirmations help to heal unresolved issues. We are involving the whole brain and allowing the body to access its own divine healing wisdom. Your intention is to bring the intensity of the feeling to still-point (0), where you feel calm, peaceful and at ease. Some feelings are so ingrained in the system that they need more work. Make a note in your journal and work every day until you reach still-point. You can also use the other acupoints for deep work.

At the end of each day, evaluate how your day went and the times when you felt stressed, irritated or negative. Take each time through the Emotional Healing Formula or make a note in your journal. Note the date and incident.

Reserve some time to catch up on your unresolved emotional load. Soul-cleansing is hard work when you start, but very soon it will become smart work and eventually no work at all! Work through as many triggers, stressors and unresolved feelings as possible. Remember that beliefs are higher up the hierarchy than feelings. Also pay attention to recurrent self-critical thoughts and any thoughts you have that reject or ridicule you or make you feel inferior. Your attitude toward life and your physical feelings should also be in this equation.

You are learning to pay attention and become a better observer of yourself. You are connecting more and more to the 'I', and this is a spiritual journey! As you go along, you will know the Emotional Healing Formula by heart and always have it available for any occasion.

Important Warning

Never let the Emotional Healing Formula become just an intellectual exercise, just a script you read. It should involve your mind, body, soul and spirit. You can say it out loud or silently, it doesn't matter. Your full attention should be on it.

Once in a while you will still have feelings that are difficult to verbalize. The labels are not really important. Just grade the intensity of the feeling from 0 to 10, and focus on the feeling of discomfort while you are working through the Emotional Healing Formula. In the next chapter we'll look at some additional tools to break through deep unresolved layers.

To end this chapter, here is a quote by an anonymous author my sister gave to me:

The Choice Is Mine

I choose to live by choice, not chance
I choose to make changes, not excuses
I choose to be motivated, not manipulated
I choose to be useful, not used
I choose self-esteem, not self-pity
I choose to excel, not compete
I choose to listen to the inner voice, not the random opinion of the crowds.
The choice is mine, and I choose to surrender to the will of the Divine Mind, for in surrendering I am Victorious.

CHAPTER 14

THE PATH TO INNER PEACE

We all basically want the same things: to feel happy, loved and successful. Not necessarily 'successful' in terms of power, money and fame, but more the feeling of having made something of your life. Unconditional love and universal love are not easy and they give us the wonderful opportunity to deep emotional healing and find the path to inner peace. Here are some ideas to help you achieve this path to inner peace.

THE FOUR CIRCLES OF INFLUENCE

1: Start with the people in your life with whom you have an intimate relationship. These may be parents, spouses, children and close family such as brothers and sisters and dear friends. *This is your inner circle.*

2: Follow with the next circle around your inner circle – people you have frequent or regular contact with such as neighbours, colleagues or members of a club. *This is your social circle.*

3: Follow with people who come in and out of your life and are either acquaintances or relative strangers. *This is your outer circle.*

4: Finally, people who have caused you harm or pain. This may include people who are in the first three circles. *This is your karmic healing circle.*

Let's look now at unconditional and universal love, then go back to these four circles of healing.

Unconditional Love

This means loving another person regardless of his or her personality, action, beliefs or behaviour. This love exists no matter what the other person does; it may be a one-way street where we let our feelings, emotions and actions flow out toward the person, without any expectations. Even when they disagree with us, abuse us, take advantage of us or never show gratitude or remorse, or even when they resent us or ridicule us – that's real unconditional love. It does not depend on any return of affection or appreciation for what we do or give.

Universal Love

Universal love means loving everyone regardless of whether we have a close relationship with them or not. They might be total strangers we know nothing of. They can differ in race, colour, socially, academically, politically and so on. That is a very high goal to achieve, and for most of us almost impossible, but certainly worth a try.

Our Karmic Healing Circle

This is the most difficult one: loving another person who has hurt us or our loved ones. It is even worse when they show no remorse or intention to change. The most intense situations are when loved ones have died and the person responsible has not received what we'd consider appropriate punishment by the authorities. That causes us to experience anger, frustration and bitterness. These very situations, however, offer the opportunity for deep healing and to discover much about ourselves. It is to be expected that confronting situations like this will cause us great discomfort. With emotional balance we can find the path to inner peace. It is always worthwhile.

The four circles of influence increase in difficulty to help us to develop unconditional and universal love. Remember: the path to inner peace starts with forgiveness and letting go of the past.

Starting with your inner circle, make a list of all the people in this circle and check which ones stress you the most. Also check to see if you can recognize any typical patterns (chains of typical reactions). Enact your healing sessions on these people, until you feel totally loving toward them. Take as much time as you need – also read further in this chapter on specific emotions and how to treat them.

When you feel completely at ease and loving with the people in your inner circle, you can move on to the people in your social circle. Here you do the same as for your inner circle, taking as much time as you need. Then work on all the people in your outer circle until you feel completely at ease and loving toward any new person you meet. Take as much time as you need.

Last but not least, go to your karmic healing circle. Read Chapter 10 on forgiveness again, then forgive each and every person in this circle, using the forgiveness and anger acupoints. Then use the Emotional Healing Formula for each person. Keep doing this until you feel completely at ease and loving when you think of them. This may take a while, but I am sure it will have a tremendous positive impact on your life. Only then can you have unconditional love for others, regardless of any pain or harm they may have caused you or your relatives. It is the easiest path to inner peace and harmony. Any time anyone causes you stress or discomfort, you will have an opportunity to heal another part of yourself. Be happy with these opportunities. In Chinese, the words for 'crisis' and 'opportunity' are the same; now you understand why: in every crisis there is great opportunity to grow and heal – welcome the crisis as the great opportunity it really is.

THE NEXT STEP ON THE PATH TO INNER PEACE

Next on the path to inner peace is working on the specific emotions and using the 14 gateways to emotional balance.

In order to heal completely, the *Chi* has to flow through all 14 meridians freely, so the whole body is regenerated. Wherever there is a limitation, discomfort or disease in our body, we should use a combination of the Emotional Healing Formula and balancing all 14 gateways while focusing on the part or organ that needs support.

The Seven Primary Emotions

The path to inner peace is achieved by integrating the seven primary emotions: Fear – Anger – Hurt – Worry – Grief – Stress – Overexcitement. There are two ways to do this: whenever we feel any of these specific emotions or related ones, we use an 'Intensity Index' to grade it from 0 to 10. Then we do the emotional reversal procedure (see Chapter 9).

After this, we need to treat all 14 gateways with the appropriate affirmations, and then undertake the Emotional Healing Formula. If your 'Intensity Index' is not yet at 0, treat the 14 gateways (acupoints) again. Treat all 14 acupoints at least once a day, and preferably twice: mornings and evenings. This will help the Chi circulate through the body and increase vitality.

Physical Problems

When someone has physical complaints, the healing can be accelerated tremendously by using a combination of the Emotional Healing Formula and the 14 gateways to emotional balance. While doing the Emotional Healing Formula, focus on the physical complaint. Immediately follow with the 14 gateways and their specific affirmations, linking them to the complaint. For example: 'I deeply love and accept myself with my fear and insecurity related to this physical condition.' This balancing is geared toward healing the past and all related incidents and conditions. So don't worry, nothing can go wrong, you cannot create a physical problem that you don't already have; you can only heal what you have.

Please refer back to pages 147–61 for our discussion about emotions and their associated images and affirmations.

SUMMARY

We are responsible for creating our own inner peace. There is no one who can do that for us. Creating discipline in your life is the only way to do this. It is a spiritual discipline because it will bring you closer to your spirit. It is an investment in time and effort, and for a lot of people this is a big turn-off. We are conditioned to believe that there are instant answers to all our problems. Watch TV and see how many illusions the smart corporations create in their attempts to get us to buy their products and services. Millions are paid to sportspeople and film stars to be associated with a product. Most of these celebrities do not care about the product or you. They are paid good money to endorse a product. It is time to wake up. There is only one way to achieve inner peace, and that's through working harder and smarter. The more you invest in yourself, the higher the return. Over time your life will become smoother and easier. You will start attracting different types of people and situations in your life. What is it worth to you, to get more out of your life? More joy, more happiness, more pleasure, more years, more quality, more life itself? What if all you have to do is spend a little bit more time on yourself? What if this investment is so cheap and yet so effective that it adds many more vital years to your life, would you do it? Of course you would. So start now; start with 15–20 minutes a day and, as you feel better and need less sleep, increase to 30 minutes each day investing in the development of spiritual intelligence and emotional balance.

What to Work On
Long-term: your circles of influence. Starting with your inner circle going to the fourth karmic circle, creating unconditional and universal love in your life.

For acute stress: respond daily to any stress from any of these circles by balancing the stress out.

Daily balancing: the seven primary emotions – balance the 14 gateways daily for optimal results.

Any physical problems, disease or discomfort: even stiffness in the muscles, menstrual cramps, problems sleeping and nightmares fall into this category. Also, post-operative complaints are important to look into.

Life issues – becoming responsible:
- forgiving all, past and present
- feeling worthy of receiving love, joy, good health

- letting go of shame, guilt, resentment and judgement
- letting go of the need to control, abuse, use power
- letting go of the need for approval, appreciation, acknowledgement
- feeling adequate facing obstacles and challenges
- loving all of God's creation and appreciating those lessons that come to us disguised as crises
- being grateful for our blessings.

Taking full responsibility for our actions, words, thoughts, beliefs and feelings means we are truly embarking on the path to inner peace. Now you have the tools, the rest is up to you. You can begin, knowing always that you cannot go wrong. These methods have been tested and perfected by more than 20,000 people, resulting in as many success stories. Yours is next. Freedom is waiting for you and inner peace is all yours.

CHAPTER 15

SYNCHRONOETICS: ATTRACTING THE FUTURE

'Noetic' is derived from the Greek word *nous*, meaning 'mind', 'intelligence' or 'ways of knowing'. The noetic sciences comprise an interdisciplinary study of the mind, consciousness and diverse ways of knowing. I have coined the word *synchronoetics* to focus our attention on the logic behind the Level 3 of manifestation, the level of synchronicity. Deepak Chopra teaches workshops on what he calls 'synchrodestiny': making the universe work for you. Synchronoetics is similar in intent: in synchronoetics one starts with cleaning up the past and finding inner peace through emotional healing. By cleaning up your past, you are also changing the information you are sending into the morphogenetic field. You are releasing layer after layer of karmic information that no longer serves you, and you are attracting new opportunities and people through a series of improbable coincidences which Deepak calls 'a conspiracy of the universe'. I could not agree more. There are many aspects to study in this new science of creating our future and attracting our desire. Some call it 'the Secret'; others call it common sense.

INTENT

Your intent has to be clear and congruent. Whatever you want, you must create a clear image of it and become totally congruent with it. Bring this image to every chakra and use the Emotional Healing Formula to clear any sabotaging beliefs, thoughts, emotions or feelings that will keep you from being totally congruent with it. Also use the emotional reversal (see page 264) to integrate it completely. Using the 14 gateways can help you to fine-tune and balance each meridian with the multi-dimensional, multi-sensorial image you have created.

- *Chosaku:* your goal must be karma-logical, free of negative karma. It should harm no one and be beneficial to your evolutionary process.
- *Detachment:* at Level 3, there is no attachment. Accept that it may never come and detach any feelings of happiness or fulfilment from your image. You must be as happy without it as with it. It should not give you greater self-esteem or make you feel better than someone else. Lovingly detach.
- *Give specific instructions to your guides or angels:* let them deal with the details. During your daily meditation, you just visualize your image and experience all the feelings of having it in your life. Keep the feelings in your day-to-day life and give the image to your guides and angels.
- *Pay attention to the signs:* the universe communicates with you in a universal language, using all possible signs and coincidences. Everything has a meaning. My agreed sign with my angels and guides is sneezing. When my partner or I sneeze, or even if someone else does, I know there is a message coming.

You can start by paying attention to your eternal moment of now. Keep your eyes and other senses open for the signs that will come. Just begin with finding out the series of coincidences that led you to this book. Next step is to find out how you can learn more; possibilities include attending a workshop or seminar, reading more books or buying an awareness-inspiring DVD or CD. Immerse yourself completely, and also study meditation. I practise primordial sound meditation as taught by instructors trained by Deepak Chopra. I also practise Qigong, which brings you to your inner core. Without a spiritual practice it can prove more difficult to experience the full benefits of synchronoetics and your magnetic powers of creation, and to attract the good things and people into your life.

Spiritual intelligence is synchronoetics, and this is the result of healing your soul. I want to share with you the story of a patient of mine and how her subconscious and Higher Self communicated. As you will see, the universe has a peculiar way of communicating with us. Everything can mean something; it is up to you to find out what the meaning is for you.

THE STORY OF ANJA

Anja looked good and her eyes were twinkling. She was 36 years old and had undergone surgery four months before and had radiotherapy for cancer in her right breast. She is an alternative health practitioner. She had seen a host of alternative practitioners and was confused by all the contradicting theories and recommendations. She showed me she was taking over 40 different remedies. 'How do you do that?' I asked. 'My partner checks me every two days, through muscle-testing, to find out what I need!' She told me that, after the surgery to remove the cancerous lump and some lymph nodes, all went very well for a while. For the past few weeks, however, she had had some swelling in her breast and in the armpit region. Also her breast was very sensitive to the touch. 'So, what have you learned from all this?' was my next question. She said that she was not quite sure. She had the feeling that before the detection of the cancer, she had been doing fine. She had been working on her emotions and had changed a lot of things in her life. She was feeling more balanced, happy and then, just when all was going right, she got cancer. A clairvoyant she had visited had told her that there were no lessons to be learned and that this was just some old stuff she had to deal with. She was very happy with that interpretation. 'I agree with the clairvoyant about it not being a lesson,' I said. 'My opinion is that we are not here to learn any more lessons. I personally believe we are beyond the lessons stage now. I believe we already know everything; we're just not *aware* of it. Instead of embarking on the inner quest of finding our potential, we go out in the world seeking excitement, entertainment, sensation. Every time we come up against an obstacle, we start looking for the lesson behind it, still looking outside ourselves for answers instead of asking ourselves, "What am I not aware of?" It is about being aware that we are not true to ourselves, being aware that we don't want to let go, being aware of our attachments and karmic patterns. There are no lessons and we have no journey to undertake to find enlightenment. We are already enlightened; we just have to become aware of who we truly are!'

Anja was silent for a moment, letting this sink in. I asked her, 'What I want to know is, what is your body or subconscious trying to communicate to you? Why your right breast and not something else? Why now? What are you not aware of? What is happening in your life in repeated patterns that you are not able to break?'

She looked at me in amazement. She had not thought about that; she had been so preoccupied getting over her cancer.

'Let's focus on one question first,' I went on. 'Why did you insist on seeing me? You have been to over seven practitioners, the best in their fields. What do you expect I can do that they couldn't?'

'I don't know,' she replied. 'There's been a voice telling me that I had to come to you and I just couldn't get it out of my system, and besides, my partner Dan wanted me to see you, too! Then I saw you on TV [*this was a synchronoetic event*] and decided to call straight away.'

I was in my thoughts for a moment, because I felt there was something synchronistic at work here; normally I am so busy that people have to wait at least six months to get an appointment with me. I went to my assistant to find out how Anja had got an appointment so quickly. My assistant replied, 'She rang just seconds after someone had cancelled an appointment, and because I knew that her partner Dan is a very good friend of yours, I decided to give her the appointment.'

Another peculiar thing was that Dan's first wife had died of breast cancer. I knew that I needed to speak to Dan about why he was attracting this into his life. Meanwhile, I came back to the now and said to Anja, 'OK, let's go deeper and do some testing to find out more.' When I tested her on being open to testing and to allow me to find the cause, she was only 4 per cent congruent with this. The blocking emotion was frustration: frustration with all the things in her life she had difficulty accepting. When I tested what the most frustrating issue was, it came out that it was having had to undergo surgery. A part of her could not accept the fact that here she was, a holistic practitioner, and she'd had to resort to traditional medicine. Then we went to check more about the right breast: it had to do with her masculine side and with male partners. When I asked more specific questions, it was revealed that she had had a troubled relationship with her father (who, by the way, was deceased) and with all her previous and current relationships with men. Her father had always been making promises that he couldn't keep: the conclusion she'd drawn from this was that men were not to be trusted and, simultaneously, that she was not loveable enough. She also lost the trust in her masculine side, including her immune system. (The immune system is part of our male aggressive side: it works like an army attacking and destroying whatever is not in harmony with the body.) Now she had created a tumour that represented her not being able to live in harmony with her masculine side and not being able to forgive her father or let go of the past. Representing her unforgiving side, the tumour had aggressively attacked her where it hurt most: her femininity.

Anja's fifth chakra was also blocked and she had difficulty expressing her inner feelings. Intimacy with men was a big issue for her. Her previous partners had all given up. Her current partner had told her that he would not give up and would not let her go. Shortly after that he'd cancelled a dinner date. That was the trigger for her immune system to break down, and two months later the tumour was discovered. She had had a preference for women doctors and healers, but by coincidence she'd heard someone talking about me, saying I was so in touch with my feminine side, and that clicked with her subconscious.

Anja was completely blown away by what came out and how everything fitted synchronoetically together. I also told her that the person who'd cancelled and whose appointment she had been given was one of the most well-known celebrities in the Netherlands, who as a result of being treated with emotional balance techniques had decided to change her life radically and had booked a two-week holiday with her husband for the first time in five years, to go to the Far East – a flight of over 16 hours (she'd been afraid of flying). The universe accommodates its children in strange ways. Anja was going to work on healing her past, forgiving her father and opening herself up to more intimacy.

MEETING DEEPAK CHOPRA

From all the hundreds of stories I know, this one is typical for the magic of synchronoetics or, as Deepak Chopra would call it, *synchrodestiny*. In case somehow you have not heard of him, Deepak Chopra is one of the foremost pioneers in sharing the old Vedic sciences, explaining them through modern quantum physics. He is the author of more than 20 books, of which several have been bestsellers. He has also coached several celebrities when in distress. He travels all over the world sharing his message: that we can become the true creators of life instead of the victims of the collective conspiracy. In 1995 I first heard of Deepak in the Netherlands through a friend of mine, Ralph Bakker, who was the first to bring Deepak to the Netherlands. Ralph and I are the co-authors of the book, *Vitality Medicine*. This was my first book and it was a very difficult task to write it. It took me more than nine months to finish my part of the book. I thought there must be another way, and when Ralph told me about Deepak and how many books he had written, I decided to ask him for his advice. I did it in a different way than one would expect: I went into meditation. At that time I was experimenting with contacting spiritual guides and asking them for advice. When I asked them how Deepak could write so many books, they told me (I was seeing and hearing this in my head), 'Why don't you ask him yourself?' The moment they said that, Deepak appeared in front of me. My first observation was of his calmness and serenity; he was open and very down to earth. I asked him the question. He smiled patiently, as if talking to a young student (which of course I am) and said, 'You have to trust your Divine Creative Force. Just allow it to happen, do not force anything. Trust that it will happen in just time.' As soon as that was said, he disappeared, with some last words: 'I am looking forward to meeting you again!' I was completely mesmerized. Was I just imagining this or was it real? I went out and bought four books by Deepak Chopra and put them on my desk as a reminder of this unique experience. Some months later I had written two more books, each in the record time (for me) of a couple of weeks.

A few years later, in late 1997, I received a mailing about Deepak's workshops. This one was called 'Seduction of Spirit' and was to take place in Goa, India: a one-week meditation retreat with Deepak Chopra to be held in March of 1998.

I looked at the brochure and wished I could go, but I did not have the time or the financial resources. I had heavily invested in a new enterprise in the Netherlands and my bank account was deeply in the red. I threw the brochure into the bin. Two days later my sister took out the bin, but when it came back the brochure was still stuck to it. I took it out, crunched it into a ball and played 'bin basketball' with it: after three misses I managed to get it in the rubbish basket. Shortly after that, my two boys Sunray (nine) and Joey (seven) were in my office and, as usual, playing and running around. After they left I found the brochure on my desk. All of a sudden I got the message: my guides were trying to tell me something. I went again into a guided meditation and I received the message: 'You have to go to India.' 'Why?' I asked. 'To meet Deepak Chopra.' 'Why all the way to India?' The answer was: 'Just do it!' So, here I was, totally in distress. If I went to India, I wanted my partner to go as well. We were low on cash but, after some debate, we decided to go using my frequent flyer miles. On 26 February we left for Mumbai. We arrived in Goa on 28 February, a Saturday, around noon. It was a very long flight all the way from Florida. On Sunday 1 March, we started with an introduction into 'primordial sound meditation'. My instructor was Mallika, a very nice and good-looking young Indian woman. She was very soft-spoken and gave me my special mantra (these are specially formulated for each individual based on their time and date of birth). We talked a little bit and she told me she was Deepak's daughter. I smiled and said, 'You're the first sign.' She did not understand, nor did I bother to explain. I had asked for some signs that this was all that was supposed to be and that all was going to plan on Level 3 of consciousness.

'Do you think there is a chance I could speak with your father privately for a few minutes?' She answered, 'There is a good chance, as he is not always busy when he is doing these seminars.' I left excited and happy with this good start. On Monday we did some yoga in the morning and a group meditation and, in the afternoon, Deepak introduced the group to some special *sutras*. It was very interesting finally to see him and he seemed exactly as in my meditation from a few years before. The day flew by and was very enjoyable and rewarding. That evening, during dinnertime, a friend of mine, Lucy Romero, a psychologist and meditation instructor from Mexico, came running up to me. She said, 'Deepak's wife, Rita, has had an allergic reaction to something and nobody can help. I told them you can cure her!' I was shocked; this was not the sign I'd expected (I didn't fully realize then that you should not expect anything in particular). I agreed to see her and to see what I could do. After the workshop I went to my room with my partner. She had packed some ointments together for sunburn, after-sun, mosquito repellent and she had also a homeopathic cream for allergies which had been packed along with the rest 'by accident'. I took it with me when I went to see Rita. She was calm and showed me the area where she was reacting in her neck. I used the muscle-test and the ointment was exactly the right remedy for her. This was a one-in-a-million chance that left me totally flabbergasted. I actually started to doubt myself and wanted to do a full emotional work-up on her, but a voice in my head said the words, 'Trust, it's all OK and part of the plan!' So I relaxed and gave her the tube with instructions, and told her if there were no change to let me know. On Tuesday I saw her again around lunchtime; she was doing much better and felt relieved. On Wednesday, after the workshop, I went to talk with Mallika, who was sitting behind a desk at the rear of the workshop-room. I had just received a fax from a friend of mine, Dr Rosa Moreschi from Italy, to ask me if I could invite Deepak to Italy to do a lecture for our Italian medical group. Each year we held a special event and the doctors trained by me would bring their patients to this workshop. Together we would work on our emotional issues. She said they would like Deepak to come and speak. Just as I was asking Mallika if it would be possible to meet her father, Deepak and Rita entered the room. 'Why don't you ask him yourself?' Mallika said, smiling, and pointed at Deepak and Rita, who at that moment reached me as Rita said, 'Deepak, let me introduce you to Dr Roy, who helped me with my allergy.' Deepak shook my hand and thanked me. 'Is there anything I can do for you?' he asked. I smiled and said, 'Yes, I would like five to 10 minutes of your time. Would that be OK?' 'What about lunch tomorrow?' Deepak replied. On 5 March, we had lunch together.

This lunch would go on to have a tremendous impact on the rest of my life. Beginning in 1999, I was a guest speaker at several of Deepak's workshops, and his organization hosted a number of my 'Inner Peace Healing' workshops. I also did a four-day workshop with him in Rome and learned a lot just by observing him.

BEGIN NOW

It all starts now: listening to the universe and your body. Right now the universe is telling you it's time to begin with your journey to inner peace and healing. Until that journey is started, nothing else is really important. It is all up to you! Do you love yourself enough to discover who you truly are? If you've come this far, I know the answer is *yes* and right now a cosmic chain-reaction of synchronistic space-time events is starting, which may lead to us meeting somewhere in cyberspace. I wish you vibrant health, unconditional happiness and inner peace!

Namaste,

Roy

Curaçao, 19 March 2010
(12 years after this book was written for the first time)

AFTERWORD

NOTES TO PONDER

Read this list every day for the next three weeks: it will change your life. After reading it, meditate for 15 minutes to allow all this information to sink in.

- Incorporate challenge into every aspect of your life to guarantee aliveness. If you don't make your life interesting, your mind will do it for you.
- What society calls right and wrong, and moral and immoral, is not necessarily true.
- When you're upset about the way it is and do nothing to change the situation, you are choosing to allow it to continue.
- Other people are a mirror for you, because the traits you respond to in others, you recognize in yourself.
- All manifestations begin with an idea. Ideas and experiences create beliefs which, in turn, create reality.
- Awareness is measured by how much you let yourself know of your own truth.
- We are all reflections of our own thoughts. So unhappiness and failure are self-inflicted while happiness and success are self-bestowed.
- If you want to understand something or someone, you must observe without criticizing.
- Whatever you can conceive and believe, you can achieve, as long as your desires are realistic and do not conflict with the free will of others.
- What you deny others will be denied to you.
- Love others as they would like to be loved, treasuring their uniqueness while accepting them as they are.
- The greatest gift you can give another person is to be all of who you are.

- In your heart you know the right thing to do at each moment in time.
- You can detach from the chaos in your life by refusing to choose to control the outcome.
- Your viewpoint determines how you react to life. You're always free to choose a different viewpoint.
- You need difficult people in your life to provide opportunities to test your resistance to what is.
- What your mind has created, your mind can change.
- The primary reason people are not as happy or fulfilled as they desire to be is because they do not know exactly what they want.
- Simplicity is one of the key secrets of wellbeing.
- Refuse to make a choice based upon the expectations of others. Instead, act in ways consistent with your purpose.
- Imagination is more powerful than willpower. Change begins with imagination.
- Practise being centred; physically relaxed, emotionally calm, mentally focused and spiritually aware.
- Practise persistence. Increasing self-discipline is a matter of building the strength not to give up.
- Very little in life is really important, so separate what is from what isn't and respond only to what is.
- What you resist in other people, other races, other lifestyles, you become, if not in this life, in the next.
- In life you experience what you are deeply convinced is so.
- Value being who you are more than being accepted.
- You are body/mind/spirit, not body and mind and spirit. What your mind doesn't handle, your body will try to resolve, draining spiritual energy in the process.
- Suffering is also the source of your awakening.
- When you're upset or life isn't working, become an 'observer' by mentally filtering the situation through the observer's detachment.

285

- You will never succeed beyond the size of your vision. So think big.
- The universe will support your clearest desires.
- Pursue your desires with no indecisiveness whatsoever. This assures you of getting what you want.
- You will achieve self-actualization momentarily, lose it and then go after it again. Eventually it sinks in.
- Never use fear as a justification for avoiding life.
- Never do things you will have to karmically punish yourself for.
- Never do anything that causes you to lose self-esteem.
- Forgive others, knowing that forgiveness is a selfish act you do for yourself to elevate karma and improve the quality of your life.
- Wake up.

RECOMMENDED READING AND RESOURCES

Nick Bunick, *In God's Truth* (Hampton Roads Publishing Company, 1998)

Luke Chan, *101 Miracles of Natural Healing* (Federation of Alcoholic Residential Establishments, 1996)

------, *Secrets of the Tai Chi Circle* (Benefactor Press, 1993)

Deepak Chopra, MD, *Quantum Healing* (Bantam Books, 1990)

------, *Perfect Health* (Bantam Books, 2001)

Larry Dossey, MD, *Be Careful What You Pray For, You Might Just Get It* (HarperSanFrancisco, 1998)

Dr Wayne W Dyer, *Staying on the Path* (Hay House, 2006)

Dr Meyer Friedman and Dr Ray H Rosenmann, *Type A Behavior and Your Heart* (Wildwood House Ltd, 1974)

Carolyne Myss, *Anatomy of the Spirit* (Bantam Books, 1997)

Paul Pearsall, *The Heart's Code* (Broadway Books, 1999)

Ernest F Pecci and William A Tiller, PhD, *Science and Human Transformation* (Pavior Publishing, 1997)

M Scott Peck, *The Road Less Traveled* (Arrow Books Ltd, 1990)

David Richo, PhD, *Unexpected Miracles* (Crossroad Publishing Company, 1998)

Neale Donald Walsch, *Conversations with God* (Mobius, 1997)

Recommended website: www.roymartina.com

Visit here for information on workshops, our free newsletter and free downloads. I teach workshops in several countries: check the website for upcoming ones in your locality.

Omega Healing is the name of a system I've created to help you take better care of yourself and go deeper into many of the aspects covered in this book. If you are interested, I have made a two-hour DVD called *The 9 Healing Codes of Omega Healing*. It is a good place to begin because you will see me and I can take you on a healing journey that will give you in-depth information about the art of healing coming out of my 30 years of practice as a holistic medical doctor, applying techniques that will support your body and heal your soul.

If you want to learn more about training your Autonomous Nervous System to function to its fullest potential, I've developed a series of 12 audio-sessions of 45 minutes each that are precisely formulated to target your subconscious mind. These Omega Healing sessions can even be listened to while sleeping.

Last but not least, as part of the healing system I developed a series of remedies made with pure power of intention: chanting, shamanistic rituals, symbols, prayer and sacred mantras to create a healing effect that is much more profound than just what we get with homeopathy, flower essences or herbs. If you are interested you can download a free booklet from my website and study what would be most suitable to help you to the next level of healing your soul and self-image and let go of all the negative karma that is holding you back.

If you have the opportunity to attend one of my trainings or workshops, you will not only enjoy yourself but you will learn practical healing techniques that will be part of your *soul-healing toolbox*. These tools will help you have a better journey on the way to your soul's destiny. I enjoy simplifying the most complex information and making it digestible for everyone. My sense of humour will make you smile and often laugh out loud. I do not take life seriously and my motto is simple: *lighten up!* I believe that the path toward enlightenment is about becoming lighter and travelling lighter while letting go of past addictions and attachments.

You can find a great deal of fun and free stuff on my website and you are free to choose what feels right for you.

Hay House Titles of Related Interest

Cellular Awakening,
by Barbara Wren

Chakra Clearing,
by Doreen Virtue

Feeding Your Demons,
by Tsultrim Allione

How Your Mind Can Heal Your Body,
by David R. Hamilton, PhD

Matrix Reimprinting,
by Karl Dawson and Sasha Allenby

The Power of Intention,
by Dr Wayne W. Dyer

Shift Happens,
by Robert Holden

SuperCoach,
by Michael Neill

You Can Heal Your Life,
by Louise L. Hay

Do you want to discover more of life with Dr Roy Martina?

Check out his website for more information about his workshops, CDs with guided meditations, DVDs and bio-energetic remedies, all personally developed by Dr Martina.

To get a taster, visit the website
to download his
- FREE eBooks,
- FREE guided meditations,
to subscribe to his
- FREE newsletter.

In life some good things
are for FREE.

www.roymartina.com

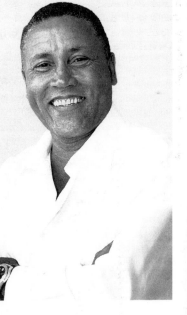

Omega Healing Training:

Being Healthy & Happy & Free is your birthright

Omega Healing is a revolutionary new method developed by Roy Martina, MD. This method is the result of 30 years of medical experience and research in the areas of vitality, peak performance, success and health.

Emotional Balance is a key part of Omega Healing

Roy Martina discovered that emotional traumas, negative beliefs, toxins, self-sabotage and conflicts will lead to deterioration and weakening of the immune system, eventually causing illness and exhaustion. The essence of Omega Healing is to create self-responsibility, stimulating the body's innate self-healing ability, so you can be your own coach and replace negative beliefs with health-promoting and vitality-enhancing ones.

Omega Healing Training by Roy Martina
Roy Martina has put his ideas into an intensive training. During the Omega Healing Training you will learn powerful tools that can enable you to eliminate subconscious sabotage mechanisms and blockages. You will understand how your beliefs affect your reality. With the Omega Healing techniques you will learn to identify the underlying destructive mechanisms and permanently remove these from your system. These techniques are very effective in the field of healing, but also offer a helping hand with other issues, including weight problems, difficult relationships or handling your finances successfully. Omega Healing addresses these problems at the root.

Find out more about our Omega Healing Training at **www.roymartina.com**

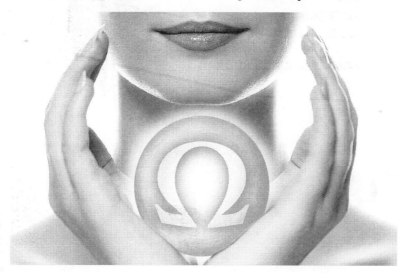

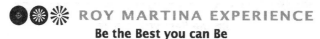
ROY MARTINA EXPERIENCE
Be the Best you can Be

JOIN THE HAY HOUSE FAMILY

As the leading self-help, mind, body and spirit publisher in the UK, we'd like to welcome you to our family so that you can enjoy all the benefits our website has to offer.

 EXTRACTS from a selection of your favourite author titles

 COMPETITIONS, PRIZES & SPECIAL OFFERS Win extracts, money off, downloads and so much more

 LISTEN to a range of radio interviews and our latest audio publications

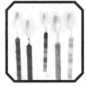 **CELEBRATE YOUR BIRTHDAY** An inspiring gift will be sent your way

 LATEST NEWS Keep up with the latest news from and about our authors

 ATTEND OUR AUTHOR EVENTS Be the first to hear about our author events

 iPHONE APPS Download your favourite app for your iPhone

 HAY HOUSE INFORMATION Ask us anything, all enquiries answered

join us online at **www.hayhouse.co.uk**

 292B Kensal Road, London W10 5BE
T: 020 8962 1230 E: info@hayhouse.co.uk